Menopause Survival Handbook:

A Complete Guide To Navigating Menopause, Managing Symptoms, Embracing Change, And Thriving Beyond Midlife!

By: Avery Rodriguez

Copyright © 2024 by Avery Rodriguez.

Disclaimer

This book is intended solely for informational purposes and is not a substitute for medical advice, diagnosis, or treatment. If you have any questions or concerns about menopause, hormone therapy, or any other health issue, it's important to consult a healthcare professional such as a gynecologist or endocrinologist. Never delay or disregard seeking competent medical advice because of anything you've read in this book.

While every effort has been made to guarantee the material's correctness, it's important to remember that medical knowledge and recommendations develop with time. The author and publisher offer no explicit or implied assurances as to the completeness, timeliness, or accuracy of the contents of this publication. Still, we are committed to keeping you informed about the latest developments. The author and publisher disclaim all duty for mistakes or omissions in this book's contents and the use or reliance on them.

This book's personal stories and experiences are unique to the individuals discussed. It's important to remember that everyone's menopausal experience is unique, and the outcomes of any therapies or lifestyle modifications mentioned in this book may differ.

For any questions about the medical conditions or treatments discussed in this book, it's crucial to consult your doctor. This book is not a replacement for personalized medical advice and treatment from your physician.

Acknowledgments

Writing this book was a journey, like menopause itself, full of surprises, challenges, and growth opportunities. It would not have been possible without so many amazing people's help, encouragement, and advice.

First and foremost, I want to express my profound gratitude to the women who shared their personal stories with me. Your unique experiences, filled with honesty and vulnerability, have enriched this book and become an integral part of its narrative. I really appreciate how you contributed.

Thank you to my family and close friends for your patience and understanding as we worked late nights and long hours to bring this book to life. Your support kept me going, even when I felt like I was out of gas (or maybe I was just having another hot flash!).

Special appreciation to the healthcare professionals and experts who generously shared their ideas and recommendations. Your invaluable experience and insights were crucial in ensuring the accuracy, balance, and usefulness of the content in this book. Your contribution is deeply respected and appreciated. You are the unsung heroes of menopause, and your work is invaluable to us all.

I'd also like to recognize the many women who came before us and faced menopause without the access and information we have now. In the face of a journey that was often misunderstood and underappreciated, your courage and resilience made it possible for works like these to exist. Your strength inspires us and empowers us to continue this important conversation.

Finally, I want to thank my readers for allowing me to join their journey. Whether you're just starting the menopausal journey or have already made it through, your role in this book is crucial. I hope this book provides you with information, reassurance, and a little bit of humor along the road.

Much appreciation,

Avery Rodriguez

Menopause Survival Handbook.

Copyright © 2024 by Avery Rodriguez. _______________________________________ii

Disclaimer____ iii

Acknowledgments ____ iv

What People Are Saying About This Book… ____________________________________ xiv

Introduction: The New Adventure begins. ___________________________________1

Why This Book? ____ 1

We're In This Together: My Menopause Journey. ______________________________ 3

How To Use This Book - A Guide To Surviving Your Menopause Journey: ___________ 5

Menopause Around The World: Understanding Cultural Perspectives. ______________ 9

Part 1: Understanding Menopause____14

1. What is Menopause?____15

The Fundamentals: Why Am I Sweating For No Known Reason?_________________15

The Exact Science Behind It: Hormones, Ovaries, And All That Jazz! ______________17

The Ultimate 12-Month Countdown: Menopause Becomes A Reality. ____________18

Why Does Menopause Occur?____19

Checklist: ____21

Action Plan: ____21

2. The 3 Phases of Menopause. ____23

1. Perimenopause: The Roller Coaster Ride You Didn't Sign Up For! ______________23

2. Menopause: The Ultimate Finale—But Not Really. ________________________26

3. Postmenopause: After The Party Ends. __________________________________28

Late-Onset Menopause: ____30

Early And Premature Menopause: When It Happens Too Soon. __________________31

Checklist: ____35

Action Plan: ____ 35

3. Menopause 101: Common Symptoms Explained. _____________ 37

Are Night Sweats And Hot Flashes The New Reality? ___________ 37

The Mystery Of Disappearing Periods. _______________________ 39

Mood Swings: Why Am I Feeling Like I'm 15 Again? ___________ 40

Sleep Problems: Counting Sheep Doesn't Cut It. ______________ 41

Vaginal Dryness: Let's Talk About It, Because No One Else Is! ___ 42

Libido: Where's My Sexy Gone? _____________________________ 43

The Bulge Battle Starts With Weight Gain. ___________________ 44

Brain Fog: Where Did My Keys And Mind Disappear To? ________ 45

Skin And Hair Changes. ____________________________________ 46

Bone Health: Learning About Menopause And Osteoporosis. ____ 47

Heart Health: Menopause And Cardiovascular Risks. __________ 48

Checklist: ____ 50

Action Plan: ____ 50

4. What Brings About These Symptoms? _____________________ 52

The Estrogen Exodus: Your Body's Great Migration. ___________ 52

Appreciating The Domino Effect: How One Hormone Affects Everything! _________ 54

The Function of Progesterone: Why It Matters And What Happens When It Declines? _______________________________________ 56

Testosterone in Women: The Lesser-Known Hormone and Its Effects. _______ 57

Checklist: ____ 59

Action Plan: ____ 59

Part 2: Navigating the Menopause Maze ____________________ 61

5. Menopause Nutrition. __________________________________ 62

Menopause Survival Handbook.

The Function Of Diet In Menopause: How Your Food Affects Your Emotions. _______ 62

Key Nutrients For Menopausal Health. _______ 63

Plant-Based Estrogen: Phytoestrogens and Their Effects. _______ 65

Foods To Embrace: Building A Menopause-Friendly Diet. _______ 66

Foods To Avoid: Those That Could Make Conditions Worse. _______ 68

Hydration: Drinking Your Way To Improved Wellness. _______ 70

Vitamins And Their Function: Negotiating The Supplement Aisle. _______ 71

Meal Planning And Recipes: Practical Advice For Eating Well. _______ 72

Menopause-Friendly Food List. _______ 73

Breakfast Menu Options. _______ 73

Lunch Menu Options. _______ 77

Dinner Menu Options: _______ 81

Ideas For Snacks: _______ 86

Dessert Menu Options. _______ 88

Checklist: _______ 91

Action Plan: _______ 92

6. Exercise And Physical Activity During Menopause. _______ **94**

Why Exercise Matters. _______ 94

Types Of Exercise: Strength Training, Cardio, Flexibility, And Balance. _______ 96

Developing A Workout Plan: Tailoring Exercises To Your Needs. _______ 98

Bone Health: Strengthening And Protecting Your Bones. _______ 99

Engage In Cardiovascular Exercises For A Healthy Heart. _______ 101

Exercises For The Pelvic Floor: Building The Foundation. _______ 102

Yoga And Mind-Body Practices: Embracing Calm Through Movement. _______ 103

Overcoming Obstacles To Exercise. _______ 104

Checklist: _______ 107

Action Plan: ___________________________________ 107

7. Lifestyle Changes That Will Make A Difference During Menopause. ___________ 109

How To Deal With Stress: Specific Yoga And Meditation Techniques To Stay Calm. _ 110

Sleep Hygiene: Creating A Sleep-Friendly Environment. ___________ 114

Checklist: ___________________________________ 119

Action Plan: ___________________________________ 119

8. Hormone Replacement Therapy (HRT). ___________________________ 121

What Does HRT Mean? ___________________________ 121

What Are The Benefits And Drawbacks? - Is This Appropriate For You? ___________ 123

Personal Stories: Actual Decisions, Real Women. ___________ 125

Different Types of HRT Treatment. ___________________ 127

The Risks and Controversies: Separating Fact from Fiction. ___________ 128

Checklist: ___________________________________ 133

Action Plan: ___________________________________ 133

9. Non-Hormonal Treatments. ___________________________ 135

Drugs And Supplements: Navigating The Pharmacy Aisle. ___________ 135

Vaginal Moisturizers And Lubricants: Preserving Comfort. ___________ 138

Acupuncture, Aromatherapy, And Other Mind-Body Techniques. ___________ 140

Cognitive Behavioral Therapy (CBT): A Mental Health Symptom-Relief Tool. ___________ 142

Which Dietary Supplements Should One Try? ___________ 147

Final Thoughts: Finding Your Way Through the Menopause Maze. ___________ 150

Checklist: ___________________________________ 151

Action Plan: ___________________________________ 151

10. What's True About Alternative Therapies? ___________ 153

What Does and Doesn't Work for Herbal Remedies? ___________ 153

The Controversy Over Bioidentical Hormones. 157

The Truth About Acupuncture And Other Holistic Approaches. 158

Phytoestrogens: Plant-Based Estrogens And Their Effects. 161

The Role of Essential Oils: Can Scents Make A Difference? 163

Checklist: 168

Action Plan: 168

11. Menopause And Your Sexual Health. **170**

Rediscovering Intimacy: How Menopause Affects Your Sex Life. 170

Sexual Confidence: Embracing Your Body And Desires. 173

How To Make Your Relationship With Your Spouse Stronger. 174

Pelvic Floor Health: Building A Stronger Base. 176

Checklist: 178

Action Plan: 179

Part 3: The Emotional Side Of Menopause **180**

12. How Menopause Makes You Feel. **181**

The Emotional Roller Coaster. 181

Why Do I Cry During Commercials? 182

How To Cope. 183

How To Deal With Anxiety: It's Not Just In Your Head. 184

Embracing The Mood Swings: Laughing (and Crying) Through It All 186

Depression And Menopause: How They Affect Each Other. 188

Self-Compassion: A Powerful Tool In Your Arsenal. 190

Final Thoughts On Self-Compassion: 192

Checklist: 193

Action Plan: 193

13. Self-Care And Compassion. 195

Taking Time For Yourself: You Deserve It. 195

Why Mental Health Is Important: Getting Help When You Need It. 196

Humor As A Coping Mechanism: Finding The Funny Side Of Hot Flashes. 197

Stay Calm During Menopause. 200

The Power of Nature: Why Being Outside Is Good for You. 201

Checklist: 202

Action Plan: 203

14. Relationship During Menopause. 204

Talk To Your Partner. 204

Getting Support During Menopause. 205

Family Dynamics: Explaining Menopause To Kids And Loved Ones. 207

Dating And Menopause: Finding Romance During Midlife Changes. 208

Building A Support System: Finding Your Menopause Network 210

Checklist: 211

Action Plan: 212

15. Menopause And Career. 213

Workplace Challenges: Navigating Menopause At Work. 213

How To Talk To Coworkers: Breaking The Silence. 216

How To Balance Your Health And Career: Strategies For Success. 217

How To Make The Workplace More Supportive. 219

Checklist: 220

Action Plan: 220

Part 4: Life Beyond Menopause 222

12.   The Postmenopausal You. 223

Getting Used To The New Normal: What To Expect Going Forward. ___________ 223

Health Considerations: Taking Care of Your Bones, Heart, and More. ___________ 225

Finding Joy And Purpose: It's Time To Focus On You. ___________ 226

Redefining Beauty And Aging: Getting Older With Grace. ___________ 228

Reinventing Yourself: Discovering New Passions And Hobbies. ___________ 229

Checklist: ___________ 231

Action Plan: ___________ 232

17. Dispelling Menopause Myths. ___________ **233**

Debunking Common Misconceptions: What You've Heard vs. What's True. ___________ 233

The Cultural Perspective: How Different Cultures View Menopause. ___________ 237

Menopause In The Media. ___________ 238

Historical Views on Menopause: How Our Understanding Has Evolved. ___________ 241

Checklist: ___________ 244

Action Plan: ___________ 244

18. A New Beginning: Embracing the Next Chapter ___________ **246**

Rediscovering Yourself. ___________ 246

Old Age And Wisdom: What Menopause Teach Us About Living. ___________ 248

How To Have The Best Life Postmenopause. ___________ 249

Travel And Adventure: Exploring the World with New Eyes. ___________ 251

Legacy And Reflection: Leaving Your Mark. ___________ 253

Checklist: ___________ 255

Action Plan: ___________ 256

Conclusion: You've Got This! ___________ **259**

Reflecting On Your Menopausal Journey: The Woman You've Become. ___________ 259

A Final Note: Celebrating Your Strength and Resilience. ___________ 261

Finally, You Can Do This! _____ 263

Helpful Links And More Reading. _____ **264**

Where to Find Out More: _____ 264

Recommended Health And Wellness Practitioners: Finding The Right Help. _____ 266

Documenting Your Menopause Journey. _____ 268

Menopausal Journaling Prompts. _____ 269

A Guide to Some Of the Good Products for Menopausal Women. _____ 276

About the Author. _____ **279**

Sharing My Story: My Journey Through Menopause. _____ 279

What People Are Saying About This Book...

A Lifeline for Women in Midlife.

"I cannot convey how much this book has helped me! The Menopause Survival Handbook does more than simply provide knowledge; it also serves as a reassuring, relevant guide to the most difficult stage of life. I was feeling overwhelmed by my symptoms, but after reading this, I discovered practical ways for regaining control. The personal stories make you feel as if you're talking to a friend who has gone through everything. A must-read for women experiencing menopause!" — *Mia Wilson., 48, New York.*

Empowering and Informative.

The book is divided into eighteen comprehensive chapters, each focusing on a different aspect of menopause, from understanding the stages to maintaining mental wellness. Each chapter is jam-packed with advice, recommendations, and techniques. I really loved the actual methods in each section — this isn't simply a theory but a practical manual. If you are going through menopause or know someone who is, this book will provide you with information and confidence." — *Chloe Johnson., 52, California.*

Practical, Compassionate, and Realistic.

"I've battled with hot flashes, mood swings, and restless nights for years, but after reading this book, I finally felt understood. The author explains everything so clearly that I felt as if I were receiving advice from a trusted friend. The suggestions are simple to apply, and I can immediately notice a change in my physical and mental well-being. This book provides the tools you need to accept the menopausal journey, and it's written with a sympathetic, personal touch." — *Megan Davis., 50, Texas.*

A Must-Have Resource for Every Woman.

"Initially, I felt uneasy because I believed that no book could accurately reflect the ups and downs of menopause. But this one does everything. The 'Menopause Survival Handbook' covers everything, including hormone replacement treatment and stress management. I feel like I've regained control of this often-overlooked stage of life, and it's comforting to know I'm not alone in this. This book certainly provides something for any woman experiencing menopause! Don't wait, get your copy today and start your journey to empowerment." — *Scarlett Brown., 46, Florida.*

Menopause Survival Handbook.

A Perfect Blend of Facts and Empathy.

"This book provides the ideal balance of factual guidance and emotional encouragement. I like how the author described her own experiences with menopause, which made me feel more understood and less alienated. The tools and practical ideas are excellent, particularly the journaling prompts and activities. It's not simply a guide; it's a partner during this life shift!" — *Sophia Reed., 53, Illinois.*

Not Just Another Menopause Book.

"I've read a lot of menopausal literature, but this one stood out. The Menopause Survival Handbook differs in that it treats menopause as a life-changing experience. It covers physical and mental difficulties, and I appreciate how the author encourages us to accept change rather than dread it. If you're going through menopause, you'll need this book. — *Stella Bennett., 49, Colorado.*

Uplifting and Inspiring.

"Finally, a menopausal book that isn't depressing! I found the passages on finding pleasure after menopause and redefining beauty to be particularly encouraging. The author writes with wit and kindness, and it's evident that she wants her readers to survive and flourish throughout menopause. "A fantastic read!" — *Emma Clarke., 51, Pennsylvania.*

Insightful and Full of Solutions.

"The Menopause Survival Handbook is more than simply a list of symptoms to handle; it's a guidebook for making the most of this time in life. I loved the emphasis on both mental and physical well-being throughout menopause. The practical advice, ranging from stress management to sleep enhancement, has already made a difference for me. I strongly recommend this book to anybody wishing to handle menopause with greater comfort and less aggravation." — *Lily Foster., 50, Arizona.*

A Helpful and Compassionate Guide.

"What a great book! Menopause is such a personal experience, and this book does a wonderful job of addressing that while also offering practical counsel for the physical and mental challenges. I like the passages on mindfulness and the powerful tone throughout. It's like talking to someone who genuinely understands. This book is a must-have." — *Ava Brooks., 47, New Jersey.*

Supportive and Life-Changing.

"If I had a dime for every time I was told that menopause was something I had to deal with, I could have paid for this book tenfold! But truly, this book changed my perspective on menopause and provided practical suggestions that I could instantly apply. Whether I'm struggling with hot flashes, mood swings, or simply learning to accept myself again, this book is my new go-to resource!" — *Grace Cooper., 55, Ohio.*

Introduction:

The New Adventure begins.

"Menopause is your body's way of saying, 'Let's start a new chapter, and this time, you're in charge.'" — Unknown

Why This Book?

Menopause is an experience for which you are never fully prepared.

If you're anything like me, you've probably spent your entire life hearing bits and pieces about menopause — a hot flash here, a night sweat there, and maybe a joke or two about mood swings — but no one has ever sat you down and told you the whole story. You may have assumed it was something far away that only happened to "older" women, and now you find yourself in the thick of it. And the first question that crosses your mind might be, "Why has no one tipped me off about what's ahead?"

That's precisely why I wrote this book. I've been where you are, looking at a fan in the middle of winter, questioning my sanity, and wondering why my garments suddenly seemed like they were made of fire.

I wanted to create the resource I wished I had — an honest, detailed, and approachable guide.

A One-Stop Guide

Think of this book as your menopause resource, equipped with all the essentials you'll require to navigate this new phase of your life. We'll look into everything from the scientific nitty-gritty to the emotional roller coaster, nutrition tips to exercise routines, the best way to deal with hot flashes, and the sometimes awkward but necessary conversations with loved ones.

It is more than just a textbook full of facts (although there will be plenty of those). It's a chat among friends — where you may learn, laugh, and possibly cry a little, but most importantly, feel supported. You aren't the only woman going through this midlife experience, so you should be well-informed and fully prepared.

Making Menopause Manageable And Meaningful.

Another goal of this book is to change the way we discuss menopause. Let's face it: the world has not always been kind to women's health challenges, and menopause is sometimes swept under the rug or viewed as a taboo. This book is designed to shed light on the subject, dispel myths, and demonstrate that menopause is a manageable, even enjoyable, stage of life.

And believe me, there's more to it than symptoms and treatments. Menopause is also a moment of transformation, allowing you to evaluate your life and reconnect with yourself. This book helps you realize that and empowers you to face change with curiosity and courage.

We're In This Together: My Menopause Journey.

Let me start by saying you're not alone if you feel overwhelmed. I remember the exact moment I realized I was entering menopause. It was a Tuesday afternoon, in the middle of a work meeting. A sudden surge of heat rose from my chest to my forehead as if I'd stepped into an unexpected sauna. I thought I was having a panic attack, but it was my first experience with hot flashes.

From there, things got interesting. Nights evolved into a series of sweaty struggles with my bedsheets, and my emotions were, let's say, simply unpredictable. I cried during advertisements and yelled at my loved ones over the tiniest things. To top it all off, I started forgetting words in the middle of sentences, which made me feel crazy.

Does this sound familiar? If so, welcome to the club that no one wants to join, but once inside, you discover that it is filled with strong, resilient women like you.

Why I Am Here for You.

One other reason I decided to write this book is because, during the early stages of my menopause, I felt disoriented. I searched the internet for answers, but most of what I found needed to be more clinical, precise, or comforting. I needed someone to sit me down, offer me a cup of tea (or a bottle of wine), and say, "Here's what's going on, and here's how we're going to get through it together."

So, this book is your companion in the menopause journey. I'm here to guide you, share what I've learned, and assure you that it's okay to feel whatever you feel. I'll share my personal experiences, the good, the bad, and the downright embarrassment, because if we can laugh about it, we can get through it.

Keep in mind that everyone experiences menopause differently, and there is no single correct or incorrect approach to it. Your journey is personal, so take it at your own pace. Some days, you'll feel like you've got everything under control; while other days, you'll want to hide under the covers. Both are okay and part of our unique, sometimes challenging, menopausal journey.

The Power of Community.

One of the most important lessons I learned during my menopause experience was the value of community. When I began openly discussing what I was going through, I realized how many other women were going through the same thing, but no one was talking about it. We shared suggestions, tales, and laughter, which made things seem less frightening.

That is why I encourage you to connect with other menopausal women — sharing your experiences through a local support group, an online forum, or a simple conversation with your best friend, could be highly encouraging. You'll quickly learn that you're not alone and that there's a whole tribe of women who understand exactly what you're feeling.

So, let's go on this journey together. I pledge to be with you every step of the way, offering advice, making you laugh, and assuring you that you can do it.

How To Use This Book - A Guide To Surviving Your Menopause Journey:

A Book for Every Phase.

This book is designed to be amenable to your needs, allowing you to take control of your menopausal journey. Whether you're just noticing changes in your body, navigating perimenopause, or embracing postmenopause, you can skip to the sections most relevant to you. You're in the driver's seat, and reading from cover to cover is entirely up to you.

Here's an overview to help you explore:

- **Part 1: Understanding Menopause.** This part covers the fundamentals of Menopause, including what, why, and how. If you want to build a firm foundation of knowledge, start here.

- **Part 2: Navigating the Menopause Maze.** This section delves into practical advice and tactics for symptom management. From nutrition and exercise to hormone replacement therapy and alternative remedies, this is the section you look to for helpful information.

- **Part 3: The Emotional Side of Menopause.** This section explores the mental and emotional elements of Menopause. This section will be handy if you are experiencing mood swings, worry, or simply attempting to make sense of your feelings.

- **Part 4: Life Beyond Menopause.** This part focuses on embracing the next stage of your life. Here, you'll find inspiration and advice for flourishing after Menopause, from rediscovering your hobbies to living your best life.

Interactive Elements:

I've also included some interactive elements throughout the book:

- **<u>Journaling Prompts:</u>** These help you reflect on your experience. Feel free to write in the margins, grab a notebook, or even start a menopause journal to track your thoughts and feelings.

- **<u>Checklists and Action Plans:</u>** At the end of each chapter, you'll find practical checklists and action plans. These are not just tools; they are your roadmap to taking control of your menopause journey. They are meant to help you apply what you've learned and take proactive steps towards managing your menopause.

- **<u>Personal Stories:</u>** I've strategically included personal stories throughout the book, mine and those of other women who've generously shared their experiences. These stories remind you that you're not alone and that there's no one-size-fits-all approach to menopause. You'll find them italicized.

- **<u>Humor Breaks:</u>** The entire book contains moments of humor subtly sprinkled throughout. These are included to remind you that laughter can be a powerful coping mechanism, especially when dealing with the challenges menopause throws our way.

How You Can Get The Best From This Book:

You must read this book thoroughly to get the most out of it. Some days, you may want to delve deeply into the intricacies of what is happening in your body, while other days, you may only need quick advice to cool down a hot flash. This book supports you wherever you find yourself on your menopausal journey.

Remember that this book is about flourishing through Menopause, not just surviving it. So, take what you need, discard what doesn't connect, and remember you are in charge of this journey. After all, this is about you and your own menopausal experience.

Menopause Around The World: Understanding Cultural Perspectives.

Menopause is a global phenomenon, but how it is seen and treated differs by culture. While some communities accept it as a natural and even cherished period, others regard it with suspicion or discomfort. Understanding these cultural differences can not only extend our viewpoint but also bring comfort in knowing that, while Menopause is difficult, it is something that women all around the globe have faced for ages.

Western Perspectives: Menopause as a Medical Condition.

Much of Western culture views Menopause from a medical perspective. It must be handled, controlled, and sometimes silently tolerated. The focus is on symptom treatment, which is frequently achieved by hormone replacement therapy and other medical measures. The debate about Menopause in the West may sometimes appear clinical and impersonal, focused on the obstacles rather than the chances for development and transformation.

However, this attitude is gradually changing. As more women (and men) open up about Menopause, there is a rising movement to change the narrative from one of sorrow to one of empowerment. This book will contribute to that transformation by analyzing the challenges and opportunities for personal growth and regeneration that Menopause may provide.

Asian Perspectives: Spiritual and Natural Transition.

In many Asian cultures, menopause is seen as a normal phase of life and is frequently associated with spiritual development and wisdom. For instance, the Japanese call Menopause '*Konenki,*' meaning renewal years. This Japanese phrase shows that Menopause is regarded as starting afresh. It lends credence to the belief that women's roles in society change while their worth remains unaffected as they journey through Menopause.

Menopause is also viewed holistically in Chinese medicine as balancing the body's energy, *Yin* <u>and</u> *Yang*. Treatments frequently focus on restoring bodily equilibrium through nutrition, acupuncture, and herbal medicines. This method contrasts with the more symptom-focused therapies commonly utilized in the West, providing an alternate perspective that stresses balance and natural transitions.

African Perspectives: A Community-Orientated Approach.

In many African societies, menopausal women are respected and considered full of wisdom. Older women are frequently admired for their knowledge and experience, and Menopause marks the shift to this esteemed status. It is not unusual for postmenopausal women to take on leadership roles in their communities, mentoring future generations and playing an essential role in preserving cultural traditions.

In several African civilizations, menopause is accompanied by special rites and ceremonies to commemorate the change and give communal support. This community-based approach may be empowering, in sharp contrast to the frequently isolating experience of menopause in the West.

Latin American Perspectives: A Time for Liberation.

In many areas of Latin America, menopause is viewed as a point of liberation, moving away from the potential for pregnancy and shifting toward self-care and personal fulfillment. The cultural emphasis is on embracing this new phase of life with enthusiasm and positivity. Women are encouraged to focus on their health, relationships, and personal goals, seeing menopause as a chance to rediscover themselves.

Within various Latin American communities, family and networks of support play a crucial role during menopause. Women often rely on the insights of older female relatives who have experienced similar life changes, fostering a sense of continuity and shared wisdom.

Indigenous Perspectives: A Connection with Nature.

For numerous Indigenous groups, menopause is recognized as a natural event closely connected to the rhythms and cycles of the earth. This transition frequently includes a significant spiritual aspect, with rituals and practices that honor the internal changes occurring within the body.

Certain Native American tribes, for instance, hold the belief that menopause enhances a woman's spiritual capabilities. This period is seen as one for reflection, engagement with nature, and readiness to impart knowledge to others. Such views foster a deep respect for aging and an appreciation for nature, which can be grounding and empowering.

Learning from Other Cultures Expands Our Views.

Gaining insight into how different cultures perceive and navigate menopause can broaden our understanding and lead to discovering new ways to approach this stage of life. There is no singular "correct" method for experiencing menopause; the key lies in finding what suits you best. Whether through embracing spiritual elements, seeking community support, or finding comfort in medical treatments, the aim is to approach menopause with an open mindset and willingness to learn.

Let's Bring It All Together.

This book will draw on these cultural perspectives to provide a comprehensive approach to menopause. You will encounter insights and guidance informed by diverse traditions, practices, scientific understanding, and personal stories. The goal is to create a resource that assists in managing the physical symptoms of menopause while also enhancing awareness of this critical life transition.

As you explore this book, remember that menopause is a shared experience that connects women across different eras, regions, and cultures. By learning from and supporting each other, we can make this transition manageable but also meaningful and enriching. Along the way, we may even find moments of joy and laughter.

Part 1: Understanding Menopause

1. What is Menopause?

"Menopause is not a disease. It's a second spring."

— Chinese Proverb

Let's start with the basics. You're here because your body is going through some rather unexpected changes. Maybe you're getting irrationally annoyed at the sound of someone breathing or sweating like it's the middle of summer in the dead of winter. Welcome to the wacky world of menopause! Let's figure out what's going on.

The Fundamentals: Why Am I Sweating For No Known Reason?

You have probably heard about hot flashes, and perhaps you even considered them a cliché employed in TV shows to make women of a particular age seem drained — a hyperbole. Now that you are personally experiencing hot flashes, though, you understand that they are natural. Oh dear, they are no jokes.

What, then, is happening when you find yourself unexpectedly sweating profusely for no apparent reason?

The scoop is like this: Your body is moving out of its reproductive years, and your estrogen levels especially are beginning to drop. Since adolescence, estrogen has been your friend; it controls your body temperature and helps to manage your menstrual cycle. Your estrogen levels are declining, so your body's internal thermostat goes wild.

Think of your body like an old radiator: for one minute, it's heating the entire neighborhood and freezing out the next minute. Hot flashes are acting in such a sort of manner. The declining hormone levels confuse your brain — especially the hypothalamus, a small but influential part of your brain that controls your body temperature. It instantly sends your body the 'sweat' alerts to believe you are overheated. And your body receives the command, 'Sweat Now,' before we all melt! And voilà, you are ripping off every item of clothing on you and instantly fanning yourself.

Hot flashes are not the only unanticipated change that lies ahead, in any case. Just as disturbing are night sweats — hot flashes that strike you while you sleep. You might question whether you unintentionally left the heating on too high when you woke up covered in wet sheets. Your body is doing its own thing, and the heater is not getting involved in what is happening in your body.

The Exact Science Behind It: Hormones, Ovaries, And All That Jazz!

Let's get scientific a bit! But don't panic; I promise to make it logical and entertaining. Menopause is the moment when your ovaries, which have been consistently generating eggs and hormones like estrogen and progesterone for decades, start to decline in its functions. Consider your ovaries as the manufacturing line of a plant that has been running nonstop for years but is now beginning to shut down.

From controlling your menstrual cycle to preserving bone density and keeping your skin young, the hormones your ovaries generate have proven vital. But usually, in your late 40s or early 50s, your ovaries slow down as you approach menopause. They start producing fewer eggs and your periods fluctuate before ending altogether.

It could take some months to many years to transition from perimenopause to menopause. Your hormone levels will vary significantly throughout perimenopause; one day, you may feel like your old self, and the next day, you are crying over a dog advertisement. It seems like riding on a hormonal roller coaster without knowing when the experience ends. These emotional changes are a normal part of the process but can be challenging to navigate.

When your ovaries cease releasing eggs, your body stops generating the exact quantities of estrogen and progesterone. This hormone decline sets off all kinds of changes in your body, including mood swings, sleep problems, hot flashes, night sweats, and metabolic alterations.

The first fact you must take note of is that menopause is a natural occurrence in every woman's life. It's not an illness or something that needs to be 'fixed'. Your body is just entering a new era of existence. Although that presents specific difficulties, it is also a period of transformation.

The Ultimate 12-Month Countdown: Menopause Becomes A Reality.

All right, so when will you be formally in menopause?
You get into menopause when you have not menstruated for a consecutive 12 months. You did indeed read that correctly — twelve months! It seems like the longest waiting game on Earth.

Your periods may become erratic during perimenopause; you may skip a month here or there or find that your cycle gets shorter or longer. You could even believe your periods are no longer coming, only to have one unexpected occurrence when you least expected it. Menopause is not regarded as official, though, until you have gone a whole year without menstruating.

Why is the 12-month restriction in place?

Because your body might be erratic throughout this change. You could spend months without a period, only for your ovaries to choose to release one last egg, creating a "farewell" period. You may formally state you have entered menopause after you cross the 12-month milestone.

After you have gone an entire year without menstruating, then menopause has set in, and you are considered postmenopausal. At this stage, some symptoms, like hot flashes and vaginal dryness, might last for several years, but the intensity of these symptoms could start to fade. Since every woman's experience is unique, there is no one-size-fits-all solution for the duration or intensity of the symptoms. Understanding what to expect during and after menopause can help you prepare for this new phase of life.

Why Does Menopause Occur?

From an evolutionary standpoint, this is a fascinating question that leads to a deeper understanding of our species' development. Here's a fascinating fact:

Menopause, a rarity in the animal kingdom, is a unique feature of humans (and a few other species, including certain whales). While most creatures continue reproducing until the end of their lives, we are the exception.

So, why does menopause affect us? From a scientific perspective, menopause is a result of the depletion of ovarian follicles, leading to a decline in estrogen production. This decline triggers a series of physiological changes, including the cessation of menstruation and the onset of menopausal symptoms.

One of the most captivating theories is the *'Grandmother Hypothesis.'* It suggests that menopause evolved to free older women from childbearing responsibilities, allowing them to play a crucial role in the survival and well-being of their offspring. According to this hypothesis, older women who can no longer bear children can invest their time and resources in supporting their existing children and grandchildren, thereby increasing the overall reproductive success of their families. This unique contribution to the family and society is a testament to the respect and value our species places on women.

Thus, menopause is not just the end of reproductive life but also the beginning of a new function whereby your knowledge, experience, and care may mold the subsequent generation. From this vantage point, this period of life has a whole new significance. Menopause is more like entering a new chapter where your contributions may take on a different but equally vital form than it is the closing of a door.

Therefore, remember that menopause serves a function even if it seems your body is betraying you with all these abrupt changes. It is a natural process that has been part of human development for thousands of years; it is related to your crucial place in the fabric of your family and society. Understanding this can bring a sense of reassurance and comfort during this transition.

Checklist:

- ☐ Understand the basic definition of menopause and its biological processes.
- ☐ Recognize the average age range when menopause typically begins (45-55).
- ☐ Familiarize yourself with the typical symptoms and signs of menopause.
- ☐ Identify the difference between perimenopause, menopause, and postmenopause.
- ☐ Acknowledge that every woman's menopause journey is unique, with varying symptoms and timelines.

Action Plan:

1. **Educate Yourself:** Delve into the biological aspects of menopause. Understanding these processes will empower you to make informed decisions about your health and well-being.

2. **Track Your Symptoms:** Start a log of any symptoms you're experiencing, such as changes in your menstrual cycle, hot flashes, or mood swings. This will reveal the regularities that will guide you to better control your symptoms.

3. **Consult a Doctor:** If you're uncertain about entering menopause, seeking guidance from your healthcare provider is crucial. They can provide the necessary tests, such as hormone level checks, to confirm your menopausal status.

4. **Talk to Women in Your Life:** Talk to friends, family members, or colleagues who have gone through menopause to gain insights and learn from their experiences.

5. **Normalize the Conversation:** Challenge yourself to talk about menopause openly with the people around you. Doing so will reduce stigma and foster a sense of community and shared experience.

2. The 3 Phases of Menopause.

"The best part of menopause? No more periods. The worst part? Everything else is up for grabs!" — Unknown

Menopause is not a single event but a journey with distinct phases, each offering unique experiences, challenges, and surprises. Think of it as a trilogy, a roller coaster ride you didn't necessarily sign up for, but now that you're on it, it's best to know what to expect at each stage.

Let us dissect the phases: Perimenopause, Menopause, Postmenopause, and the more unusual experiences of late onset, early, and premature menopause.

1. Perimenopause: The Roller Coaster Ride You Didn't Sign Up For!

If menopause is the grand conclusion, perimenopause is the substantial build-up with surprising narrative turns. Perimenopause, the transition into menopause, can be a challenging journey, with the unpredictability of hormone levels often leading to intense emotional highs and lows. It's a time that many women find difficult, and it's essential to acknowledge and understand these challenges. Knowing that these experiences are shared by many can help you feel less alone on this journey.

What Is Happening?

Perimenopause is like your body signaling, "Changes are coming!" without providing you with details but comes with a drop in your hormone levels, particularly estrogen and progesterone, which becomes unpredictable with no apparent communication with the rest of your body. This hormonal imbalance can lead to a variety of symptoms, including hot flashes, mood swings, and sleep disturbances.

Although not in a straight, linear pattern, your ovaries begin to generate less estrogen. Your hormone levels can be as expected one day and then drop the next. Many of the perimenopause symptoms are related to this irregular hormone production.

Throughout this time, you may experience any of the following:

- **Erratic Periods:** Your usual regular menstrual cycle may fluctuate. You may have two occurrences in one month, miss a period, or have flow irregularities. Your ovaries seem to be playing a game of "will it, or won't it?"

- **Hot Flashes And Night Sweats:** Thanks to changing estrogen levels, hot flashes and night sweats are typical complaints. You could be OK for one minute and then feel like someone sparked a fire within you. Your body seems to have its internal thermostat, but it is dysfunctional.

- **Mood Swings:** Have you lately been crying at a dog food ad or yelling at someone for no apparent reason? This isn't just about you! The fluctuations in hormones during perimenopause can lead to intense emotional highs and lows that may feel overwhelming.

- **Sleep Problems:** Perimenopause can disrupt your sleep habits, whether you wake up covered in sweat or cannot sleep. The usual menopausal signs are lack of sleep and constant waking up during the night.

- **Physical Changes:** Though your diet has not altered, you may find your skin drier, your hair thinner, and you are gaining weight. This fits the hormone-driven change your body is going through.

During my perimenopause, I felt like my body was rebelling. I was generally used to being in control of my body, feelings, and life. But all felt disorganized suddenly. I would go from feeling quite good to roaring like a hurricane over something as small as a lost coffee cup.

And the hot flashes? I thought my thermostat was faulty. Night sweats caused me to change my bedding more frequently than I would want to confess to. Though it was a perplexing and demanding period, knowing that these symptoms fit a more extensive picture allowed me to negotiate it more patiently.

2. Menopause: The Ultimate Finale—But Not Really.

So, you at last hit the formal milestone: menopause, following what seems to be an eternity of perimenopause. Let us define what menopause is, though, before you begin organizing a retirement party for your ovaries.

What Is Happening?

You're formally into menopause when you haven't seen your periods in twelve consecutive months. Although it's sometimes considered the "grand finale," it's more of a change into the next chapter of life as your reproductive years end. Your body is adjusting to its new reality, and the hormonal roller coaster of perimenopause starts to level down; you are not ovulating or menstruation.

Menopause often causes common symptoms, including:

- **Consistent Hot Flashes And Night Sweats:** While some women find these symptoms lessen during menopause, others may continue to experience it for years.

- **Vaginal Dryness And Discomfort:** During this phase, lowering estrogen levels cause the vaginal tissues to become thinner, drier, and less elastic, which causes pain during sex and raises urinary tract infection risk.

- **Changes In Libido:** While some women discover their libido stays the same or even rises, others find their sexual drive declines. It's all unique.

- **Emotional Changes:** Many women still go through mood and emotional well-being changes throughout menopause, even if mood swings may become less severe than during perimenopause.

My reaching menopause seems to be anticlimactic. Having battled perimenopausal symptoms for a few years, I was anticipating a big event. Instead, it was a gentle change: I knew I hadn't menstruated in more than a year, so I was formally in menopause. There was a sense of conclusiveness even though the symptoms did not go overnight. I felt comfort in my body having discovered its new balance. I'm still fatigued, but there's a sense of accomplishment — like concluding a protracted trip.

3. Postmenopause: After The Party Ends.

Congratulations: you have sailed the storm and into the postmenopausal period! On the opposite side, though, what does life look like?

Although postmenopause offers respite from some of the more severe symptoms of perimenopause and menopause, it also brings changes and difficulties.

What Is Happening?

The day after your 12-month period of being free from menstruation, a significant milestone, marks the beginning of postmenopause. Your body has become accustomed to its new normal throughout this period and is entirely ready for the lack of its reproductive hormones.

During this phase, you might notice the following:

- **Reduced Hot Flashes And Night Sweats:** These symptoms do not always go away entirely, although they may lessen. Some women experience them for years, generally with less severity.

- **Bone Health Issues:** Your risk of osteoporosis, a disorder in which bones become brittle and more likely to break, rises when estrogen levels fall. It would be best to prioritize your bone health during this period; this implies obtaining sufficient calcium and vitamin D and performing weight-bearing activities.

- **Heart Health:** Estrogen protects the heart, so the risk of heart disease rises following menopause. Maintaining a heart-healthy lifestyle, including consistent exercise, a balanced diet, and effective stress management, is essential to minimize the risk of heart disease.

- **Vaginal And Urinary Changes:** Postmenopause may bring about symptoms like vaginal dryness, thinner tissues, and urinary symptoms. However, you can manage these symptoms effectively with hormones, moisturizers, or lubricants, providing relief and comfort.

- **Constant Emotional Changes:** Although the emotional turbulence of menopause and perimenopause may calm, some women suffer from anxiety or sadness throughout. It is essential to monitor your mental health during this phase.

Postmenopause felt like a new chapter in my life. I wasn't dealing with the same level of intensity in terms of symptoms, but there was a shift in focus.

I became more aware of my bone and heart health — two things I hadn't considered much. It was also a time to redefine what this new phase of life meant for me and to set new, inspiring life priorities. There's a sense of freedom in postmenopause and a need to stay vigilant about health. It's like I've survived the wild party, but now I must clean up and care for myself.

Late-Onset Menopause:

What happens when menopause comes later than expected?
Menopause does not strike all women in their early 50s. Some people can find themselves far into their late 50s or even early 60s before they cross the 12-month barrier. This is known as late-onset menopause, and it is standard, even though it is less prevalent.

What Is Happening?

Many factors can affect late-onset menopause, including lifestyle, general health, and genetics. Women who go through menopause later may have more estrogen exposure, which can be good in some respects — such as a lower risk of osteoporosis — but it also implies a more extended trip on the hormonal roller coaster.

You may experience the following when late-onset menopause sets in:

- **Prolonged Perimenopause Symptoms:** The signs of prolonged perimenopause encompass unpredictable menstrual cycles, sudden heat sensations, and emotional fluctuations that may persist for numerous years because of the lengthy duration of perimenopause.

- **Persistent Fertility:** Although declining as one age, one can still conceive until menopause is complete. Hence, contraception could still be required.

- **Late-onset Menopause Can Cause a Range Of Emotions.** While some women are ready to be done with the symptoms, others feel appreciative of the extra time before menopause.

Women who experienced menopause later in life have told me they typically saw it as both a gift and a curse. They endured perimenopausal symptoms longer than their colleagues, although, on the other hand, they're delighted in additional years of their normal menstrual cycle.

The main lesson of menopause is that it's about managing the journey, and there is no right or wrong timing.

Early And Premature Menopause: When It Happens Too Soon.

Menopause occurs for some women well before they have had time to consider it. The most challenging are early menopause, which typically strikes between the ages of 40 and 45, and premature menopause, which strikes at a time when many women are still contemplating or actively building their families. This early start is an unexpected turn-off on a life path meant to lead in another direction.

What Is Happening?

Premature and early menopause can occur for a variety of reasons, some of which include:

- **Genetics:** Should your mother or another close female relative go through early menopause, you also have a greater likelihood of experiencing it yourself. Family history is frequently influential.

- **Medical Treatments:** Early menopause and damage to ovaries can result from several medical treatments like radiation therapy for cancer or chemotherapy. Furthermore, oophorectomy, or surgical removal of the ovaries, will lead to premature menopause.

- **Autoimmune Disorders:** The ovaries can experience early failure when the body's immune system mistakenly attacks them due to autoimmune diseases.

- **Chromosomal Defects:** Genetic disorders such as Turner syndrome often lead to premature ovarian failure.

- **Unknown Factors:** Many times, the reason for early or premature menopause is still unclear, which leaves women with more questions than solutions.

When menopause strikes early or prematurely, the abrupt decline in estrogen might cause more severe symptoms than the gradual transition of perimenopause. Thus, women might experience the following:

- **More Severe Hot Flashes And Night Sweats:** The abrupt drop of estrogen levels can cause these symptoms to be more critical in most women.

- **Emotional Pain:** Early menopause can have a significant emotional impact, especially for women who were not ready for such a major life shift at a young age or who were intending to have children.

- **Enhanced Risk Of Health Problems:** Early menopause sufferers are more likely to have osteoporosis and cardiovascular issues since estrogen helps guard against heart disease and bone loss.

It's often recommended to consider hormone replacement therapy (HRT) to help lessen these risks until menopause happens naturally.

While I didn't personally experience early or premature menopause, I've witnessed the profound impact it can have on close friends. One friend, after months of unsuccessful attempts at conception, discovered she was in an early menopause. She described feeling like her body had betrayed her, a sentiment that resonates with many women in similar situations. The emotional toll was immense, and she had to mourn the loss of the future she had envisioned. However, she eventually found peace and a new path forward.

Women in this circumstance should allow themselves the time to process their losses. Though there is no "right" way to feel this. It is OK to be enraged, depressed, or even relieved. The secret is to ask for help — from loved ones who know what you are going through, through therapy, and from support groups.

All in all, this chapter has examined several phases of menopause, each with its difficulties and opportunities. Whether you are entering an early menopause or are just noticing the symptoms of perimenopause, knowing what is happening in your body is vital.

Knowledge is power; knowing about these phases helps you negotiate the menopausal roller coaster. Remember, millions of women worldwide are going through the same thing; together, we can find courage, resiliency, and humor in challenging situations. You are not alone on this menopausal journey.

Checklist:

- ☐ Understand the three phases of menopause: perimenopause, menopause, and postmenopause.

- ☐ Recognize the typical symptoms associated with each phase.

- ☐ Know the average timeline for each phase and how long symptoms might last.

- ☐ Identify the hormonal changes during each phase and their effects on the body.

- ☐ Be aware that some women experience early or premature menopause due to genetics, medical conditions, or treatments like chemotherapy.

Action Plan:

1. **Track Your Menstrual Cycle:** Record your periods, noting any irregularities, missed periods, or significant changes, to determine if you're entering perimenopause.

2. **Monitor Symptom Progression:** Pay attention to how your symptoms change as you move from perimenopause to menopause and into postmenopause, noting any patterns in severity or frequency.

3. **Consult Your Healthcare Provider:** If you're experiencing early symptoms or are unsure which menopause phase, you're in, schedule a check-up with your doctor to discuss your concerns and possibly run diagnostic tests.

4. **Adjust Your Health Routine:** As your body moves through different phases, consider adjusting your lifestyle, such as incorporating more bone-strengthening exercises during postmenopause, when osteoporosis risk increases.

5. **Prepare for the Long-Term:** Understand that postmenopause is a long-lasting phase and that maintaining a healthy diet, regular exercise, and mental well-being are vital to thriving.

3. Menopause 101: Common Symptoms Explained.

"Menopause teaches you to listen to your body, to slow down, and to honor the woman you are becoming." — Unknown

Menopause is like an unwelcome party guest that makes their presence known in the most unexpected ways. One moment, you're floating through life, and the next, you're wondering whether you've stumbled into a whole new universe of symptoms that no one told you of.

Let's look at the most typical menopausal symptoms because understanding what's going on may help make the transition less puzzling and more tolerable. Remember, these experiences are typical and shared by many women.

Are Night Sweats And Hot Flashes The New Reality?

Hot flashes, a well-known menopausal symptom, can be a jarring experience. One moment, you're at a conference feeling comfortable, and the next, you're engulfed in a wave of heat that feels like someone has cranked up the thermostat inside your body. These rapid bursts of heat can be overpowering, leaving you soaked in sweat and desperate for understanding and comfort.

What Is Happening?

Hot flashes occur due to a sudden drop in estrogen levels during menopause. This hormonal fluctuation impairs the body's temperature control, resulting in severe heat for a few seconds to many minutes. Night sweats are just hot flashes that occur while you sleep, frequently waking you up in the middle of the night covered in sweat.

When I started having hot flashes, I believed I had a fever. Then, they became more common — during critical meetings, while driving, and even during a romantic meal. My most common symptom was night sweats. There's nothing quite like waking up at 3 a.m., feeling like you've just run a marathon, only to find it's simply your body's new "normal" routine. The game changed when I invested in a good fan and moisture-wicking sheets. And much to my family's dismay, I may have turned down the thermostat a few degrees more than usual.

The Mystery Of Disappearing Periods.

One of the most perplexing elements of menopause is that your periods begin to play hide-and-seek. You could spend months without a period, only to have it emerge out of nowhere. Alternatively, you may experience lighter or heavier periods than usual. It's as if your menstrual cycle has chosen to have one final hurrah before retiring for good.

What Is Happening?

Perimenopause causes irregular ovulation because your ovaries produce less estrogen and progesterone. As a result, your periods will become less predictable. They may move closer or further apart, and their intensity might vary considerably. Eventually, your periods will stop completely, signaling the start of menopause.

For years, I could almost set my watch based on my cycles. Then, they suddenly became unpredicted. I would spend months without one and wonder, "Is this it?" Am I finished?" Before I knew it, my menstrual flow came back more intense than it used to be. Every bag I carried included pads and tampons in case I needed them urgently. The uncertainty was irritating, but it also seemed like a gradual goodbye to an aspect of my life that had been so predictable.

Mood Swings: Why Am I Feeling Like I'm 15 Again?

If you believed mood swings were something of the past after adolescence, think again. Menopause can rekindle those emotional ups and downs with vengeance. One minute, you're OK; the next, you're yelling at someone for no apparent reason or crying over a cat food ad.

What Is Happening?

The hormonal variations during menopause can substantially impact neurotransmitters in the brain, particularly serotonin, which is essential for mood regulation. As estrogen levels fall, chemical changes might cause emotions of irritation, melancholy, anxiety, or even wrath.

I was in tears over a wilting plant on a particularly challenging day. It wasn't just a few tears; this was full-fledged sobbing. My family had no idea what to make of it, and neither did I. It felt like being a teenager again, but with the added weight of adult responsibilities. However, I've learned to give myself grace and connect with my loved ones when feeling particularly off-balance. It's not always easy, but by identifying my mood fluctuations, I've embarked on a journey of self-discovery and growth, inspiring me to handle them better.

Sleep Problems: Counting Sheep Doesn't Cut It.

Getting enough sleep during menopause might be difficult. With night sweats, hot flashes, and the overall restlessness that comes with hormonal fluctuations, obtaining a decent night's sleep might seem like a pipe dream.

What Is Happening?

Menopause causes a decline in estrogen and progesterone production, which inhibits the body's capacity to regulate sleep. The decrease in estrogen affects the melatonin hormone, which controls sleep and wakefulness. Low estrogen levels cause problems going to sleep, remaining asleep, or waking up too early. Add night sweats to the mix, and you've got a formula for insomnia.

I used to sleep like a rock, but after menopause arrived, it was as if my internal clock were locked in "awake" mode. I used to find myself wide awake and unable to go back to sleep at 2 a.m. When I did sleep, I was frequently awakened by night sweats. I tried everything, from herbal teas to meditation applications, and while they helped slightly, it was evident that my body was adjusting to a new normal. Now, I've learned to listen to my body — sometimes, that means getting to bed early, and sometimes, it means accepting that I'll be up at 4 a.m. to catch up on my reading.

Vaginal Dryness: Let's Talk About It, Because No One Else Is!

Let's have an open conversation about vaginal dryness, a symptom that is rarely discussed but is a common experience for many women going through menopause. By normalizing this discussion, we can help each other better understand and cope with this aspect of menopause.

Vaginal dryness caused by a decrease in estrogen produces weaker, drier, less elastic vaginal tissues.

What's happening?

Estrogen helps keep the vaginal walls thick and moist. As estrogen levels decline, the tissue lining the vagina becomes thinner and consequently reduces its production of natural lubrication. This change can cause discomfort during intercourse, burning sensations, itching, and an increased risk of urinary tract infections.

I was not anticipating vaginal dryness. It surprised me since no one had brought it up in my menopausal conversations. It was more than just the discomfort during sex; it was a constant dryness that wore one out emotionally and physically. Using lubricants and moisturizers was helpful, but it also took time to see that this was a new reality. Talking more with other women about it helped me better grasp how common it was, which lessened my loneliness.

Libido: Where's My Sexy Gone?

Menopause might cause libido changes for many women. While some individuals feel their libido remains stable or even increases, others may find their sexual urges decline. Although this is a very personal experience, one thing is sure: menopause could change your perspective on and attitude toward sex.

What Is Happening?

Hormonal changes linked to menopause might affect sexual desire in several ways. Insufficient estrogen can lead to vaginal dryness, which would make sex uncomfortable or painful and hence lower desire. Libido levels may also be influenced by psychological and emotional changes linked with menopause, including mood swings, stress, and body image problems.

I will admit that for some time, my interest in sex waned. Sex felt unpleasant between the mental roller coaster I was experiencing and the physical misery of vaginal dryness. My body wasn't responding as it typically would, not that I did not love my partner. We had to learn to be more open about our wants and play around with other kinds of closeness outside of sex. It was a change, but it also unexpectedly pulled us closer.

The Bulge Battle Starts With Weight Gain.

If you have noticed your weight increasing while eating the same things and working out the same way, you are not alone. Gaining weight after menopause is a common challenge, particularly around the abdominal region.

What Is Happening?

Menopause lowers hormone levels, which changes how your body stores fat. Estrogen aids in the control of body fat distribution and metabolism. As estrogen levels decrease, fat accumulates around the abdomen instead of the hips and thighs, forming what is also known as a "*menopausal belly*." Moreover, as you get older, your metabolism slows down, which makes losing weight more difficult.

For me, the weight gain of menopause was among the most uncomfortable aspects of it. I was depressed when I started to gain weight while following my meal plan since I had always been conscious of my diet and activity. It was about how comfortable I felt in my flesh and how well my clothes fit, not only about the scale numbers. I had to reassess my approach to eating and exercise, focusing more on incredible strength training and altering my diet to include more protein and less carbs. Though it wasn't easy, I learned to treat myself better and accept that my body was changing in ways I had little influence.

Brain Fog: Where Did My Keys And Mind Disappear To?

Have you ever entered a location and found yourself unable to remember why? Alternatively, do you see defining the correct term in a conversation difficult? Welcome to menopausal brain fog, a frustrating but somewhat common condition that can make you feel as though your mind is working against you.

What Is Happening?

After menopause, brain fog is commonly linked to hormonal changes affecting the neurotransmitter levels in the brain, most especially estrogen, which affects cognitive ability. The results include memory lapses, difficulty focusing, and general mental fog. Your brain is only adjusting to fresh chemical signals; you are not losing your mind.

Brain fog was one of the most unpleasant symptoms for me. Though I had always been pleased with my great memory and multitasking skills, I began to skip meetings, misplace items, and lose focus. My brain felt as though it had gone on vacation without telling me. I started compiling more exhaustive lists and setting phone reminders to keep me orderly. Though it's not the perfect response, it helped me feel more in control.

Skin And Hair Changes.

You're not insane if you find your hair thinning or your skin is dry. Changes in your skin and hair brought on by menopause can be surprising and unsettling.

What Is Happening?

Estrogen is needed to maintain healthy hair and skin. As estrogen levels drop through menopause, your skin could get drier, less elastic, and more prone to wrinkles. Hair may fall out more regularly than usual and become thinner and brittle.

I used to have a basic skincare regimen, but I realized I had to prioritize water when menopause started. My skin appeared to cry for moisture as it became so dry. My observation of increased hair in the shower drain was also quite alarming. I finally started using less harsh hair products and invested in thicker moisturizers. It took some trial and error, but I finally found a suitable schedule.

Bone Health: Learning About Menopause And Osteoporosis.

Bone health is one of the least spoken about yet most essential aspects of menopause. Reduced bone density brought on by declining estrogen levels during menopause increases the risk of osteoporosis, a disorder in which bones weaken, and brittleness results.

What Is Happening?

Estrogen promotes bone preservation by preventing bone tissue loss. Menopause causes declining estrogen levels, which increases bone loss and may cause osteoporosis if not controlled enough. This condition makes bones more likely to break, particularly in the hips, spine, and wrist.

Until my doctor brought it up during a routine visit, I gave osteoporosis little thought. When she suggested a bone density test, I was shocked to find I could be at risk. For me, it acted as a wake-up call stressing the need for bone health before and after menopause. I started on calcium and vitamin D supplements and added weight-bearing exercises to my regimen to help build my bones. Please pay attention to this early on because it's one of those things you could ignore until it's too late.

Heart Health: Menopause And Cardiovascular Risks.

Let us now go finally to the heart. The most important cause of death in women, cardiovascular disease, increases with menopause. After menopause, the declining estrogen raises the risk of heart disease and stroke as it has protective effects on blood vessels and the heart.

What Is Happening?

Estrogen lowers cholesterol and helps maintain healthy blood vessels. While HDL cholesterol (the good kind) lowers, LDL cholesterol — the bad kind —may rise when estrogen levels drop. Along with other menopausal symptoms, including weight gain and high blood pressure, this change might increase the risk of heart disease.

At first, I didn't connect menopause with heart health; then, after learning about the risks, it became a significant worry. I started paying more attention to my diet, cutting back on processed foods, and increasing my consumption of heart-healthy foods such as fruits, vegetables, and whole grains. I also started checking my cholesterol and blood pressure levels more frequently. Take it seriously, as even little changes could significantly influence them.

Menopause brings many changes — some expected, some surprising. Knowing common symptoms and how they affect your body can enable you to negotiate this new phase of life. Remember that you are not alone; millions of women are going through the same thing, so it is essential to share our experiences and help each other through the highs and lows. Knowing what's going on and why will help you control your menopausal journey, whether it's weight gain, mood swings, or hot flashes.

Checklist:

☐ Identify any common menopause symptoms you're experiencing (hot flashes, mood swings, night sweats, etc.).

☐ Track the frequency and intensity of symptoms for 1-2 weeks.

☐ Keep a journal of how your symptoms are impacting your daily life.

☐ Consult with a healthcare professional about your symptoms for guidance on treatment or management.

☐ Consider sharing your experiences with a trusted friend or loved one for emotional support.

Action Plan:

1. **Record Symptoms:** Write down the onset, intensity, and duration of symptoms like hot flashes, night sweats, or mood swings.

2. **Regular Check-ups:** It's essential to have Regular check-ups with your healthcare professional to ensure your overall health is monitored. During these check-ups, be sure to discuss any menopause symptoms you're experiencing and consider treatment options.

3. **Lifestyle Changes:** You have the power to make a difference. Based on your symptoms, research or try lifestyle changes that could

alleviate discomfort. It could include adjusting your diet or exercise routines, empowering you to take control of your health.

4. **Support System:** It's important to share your experiences with friends or family. This can help them understand what you're going through and provide the support you need, making you feel less isolated and more understood.

4. What Brings About These Symptoms?

"Menopause isn't a curse; it's a time of transformation and renewal. Embrace it as a new phase of life, not the end of the one before."
— Unknown

Understanding the hormonal changes during menopause is like learning the script of a play. If menopause is a magnificent occasion, then hormones are the unruly guests who start the party, control the music, and finally depart without cleaning up. We need to first familiarize ourselves with the central characters in this hormonal drama — estrogen, progesterone, and testosterone — to grasp why our bodies are experiencing so many changes.

These hormones control more than we could ever know. Thus, their decline during menopause sets off a series of sensations that could feel like a roller coaster ride without brakes. But armed with this knowledge, we can take the reins and confidently navigate this journey.

The Estrogen Exodus: Your Body's Great Migration.

When it comes to menopause, estrogen is usually the star of the show — and for good reason. Since adolescence, this hormone has been your body's closest buddy; it controls your menstrual cycle and helps to keep your bones healthy, among other things. But as you get ready for menopause, estrogen starts to pack bags and gently makes its way out, leaving behind a trail of symptoms that could make you feel as though your body is betraying you.

What Is Happening?

Estrogen levels are relatively stable during your reproductive years; regular fluctuations in these levels match your menstrual cycle. Your ovaries begin to generate less estrogen as you get closer to menopause, though, and these amounts might vary considerably. Many of the menopause-related symptoms, including hot flashes, night sweats, and vaginal dryness, start with this drop and inconsistency.

More so, estrogen affects your brain, skin, bones, cardiovascular, and reproductive systems. Hence, declining estrogen level is like dragging the rug out from under all these systems at once. Your body needs to get used to a new normal, and that adjustment period may be unpleasant, to put it mildly.

I did not know what may be causing my hot flashes when they started. After speaking with my doctor, I discovered the part estrogen plays in controlling body temperature. For me, it was a flashbulb event — all these symptoms I was having immediately made sense. In a way, it seemed as though my body was experiencing a great upheaval. Estrogen had been silently maintaining balance; everything was spiraling out of control as it departed.

Appreciating The Domino Effect: How One Hormone Affects Everything!

If estrogen is the main protagonist, the other hormones are the supporting cast. Though it doesn't diminish their significance, The drop in estrogen starts a chain reaction that affects other hormones and causes the symptoms of menopause to cascade.

What Is Happening?

Understanding the interconnectedness of hormones in the body is like deciphering a complex web. When estrogen levels fall, the balance of other hormones is disturbed, especially those in the pituitary and hypothalamus, which regulate many of your body's activities like temperature control, mood, and sleep. This realization can enlighten us about the intricate workings of our bodies, making us more aware and prepared for the changes that menopause brings.

For instance, the hypothalamus helps your body keep its internal thermostat intact. The confused hypothalamus caused by declining estrogen levels might cause terrible hot flashes and night sweats. Even if you're completely comfortable, your body suddenly thinks you're overheating and trying to cool you down. This is because estrogen plays a significant role in regulating your body's temperature, and its decline during menopause can lead to these sudden and intense heat sensations.

The drop in estrogen also influences your mood. Because it changes the amount of serotonin, a neurotransmitter that controls your emotions, During menopause, this might cause mood changes, anxiety, and even sadness. You are under bodily changes and ageing stress, and your brain chemistry is changing.

Realizing the domino effect of hormonal changes is like finding the missing piece of a puzzle. Hormones always seemed to me as separate beings, each working on its agenda. But I came to see that all these symptoms — brain fog, difficulties in sleeping, and more anxiety than usual — were related. My body seemed to be a perfectly tuned machine; if one component began to break, everything else matched. This understanding can provide comfort and reassurance that what we're experiencing is a normal part of the menopausal journey.

The Function of Progesterone: Why It Matters And What Happens When It Declines?

While estrogen often takes the spotlight in menopause discussions, it's important to remember the vital role of progesterone in your body. It's not just about conception but also about regulating your monthly cycle. As menopause approaches, the decline in both progesterone and estrogen levels could lead to the emergence of symptoms.

What Is Happening?

The ovaries predominantly generate progesterone after ovulation. Every month, it helps balance the effects of estrogen and prepare the uterine lining for a possible pregnancy. When ovulation becomes erratic in perimenopause, progesterone levels can fluctuate wildly. As you cease ovulating, progesterone levels eventually drop noticeably.

One reason some women have erratic periods during perimenopause is a drop in progesterone. The uterine lining may get thicker than usual without sufficient progesterone, which would cause longer or more heavy cycles. Moreover, progesterone calms the brain; hence, reduced levels might aggravate mood swings, anxiety, and sleep problems. Other symptoms that can be attributed to the decline in progesterone include bloating, and breast tenderness.

It wasn't until my cycles started behaving strangely — becoming heavier one month, then light and spotty the next- that I began to ponder the role of progesterone. Through my research and personal journey, I understood its crucial role in maintaining hormonal balance. I discovered that progesterone was essentially the unsung hero of my menstrual cycle, quietly working behind the scenes. As it began to decline, I experienced significant consequences, particularly in my mood and sleep.

Testosterone in Women: The Lesser-Known Hormone and Its Effects.

Though at lesser levels, women also generate testosterone, sometimes seen as the "male" hormone. Your general health depends significantly on this hormone, affecting everything, including libido and energy levels. Some of the changes you might be going through during menopause might be attributed to the fact that testosterone levels can drop.

What Is Happening?

Testosterone is produced by women in their ovaries and adrenal glands. It keeps sex desire, bone density, and muscular mass intact. Your ovaries generate less testosterone as you get closer to menopause, which can cause libido to drop, muscular mass to decline, and general tiredness. The decline in testosterone can also lead to a decrease in bone density, which increases the risk of osteoporosis, and a reduction in muscle mass, which can contribute to feelings of weakness and fatigue.

Although testosterone receives less attention than estrogen or progesterone, it is nevertheless a crucial component of your hormonal balance. When testosterone levels fall, it can lead to low energy, low drive, and a loss of interest in activities that used to make one happy. These can all help to explain the general "blah" many women experience throughout menopause.

I never gave testosterone much attention until menopause arrived, and suddenly, I felt as if I had lost my mojo. My sexual desire collapsed, and my energy was low. At first, I didn't even link it to hormones — after all, testosterone was something I connected with men. However, following a conversation with my doctor, I discovered this hormone was more critical than I had thought. It was a reminder that menopause is about all the hormones interacting, or in other words, not operating as effectively as they once did, not only estrogen and progesterone.

Menopause is a complicated process in which numerous vital hormones — each of which contributes in some way to the general functioning of your body — are depleted. Knowing the "why" behind these symptoms can help you understand what is occurring in your body and empower you to regulate your experience.

Menopause's hormonal changes are natural for life, even if they might be difficult. Understanding how these hormones interact and what happens when they decrease can help you better negotiate this change and develop strategies for controlling the accompanying symptoms. Remember, this is a journey. You are not alone; millions of women are experiencing the same thing. Together, we can help each other through this new phase of life.

Checklist:

- ☐ Understand the role of estrogen, progesterone, and testosterone in your body.
- ☐ Reflect on any changes you've noticed in your energy, mood, or body.
- ☐ Research or talk to your doctor about hormone therapy options (if applicable).
- ☐ Identify any lifestyle factors (stress, diet, sleep) that may aggravate your symptoms.

Action Plan:

1. **Research Hormonal Changes:** Learn how hormone fluctuations impact your body and emotions.

2. **Monitor Triggers:** Observe if any foods, activities, or stressors worsen your symptoms.

3. **Discuss with Healthcare Providers:** Bring up any questions about hormone therapy with your healthcare provider.

4. **Self-Education:** Read trusted sources about how to support hormone balance through diet and lifestyle changes.

Part 2: Navigating the Menopause Maze

5. Menopause Nutrition.

"Menopause: shedding the old, embracing the new." - Patricia Akins

Food is not just fuel. It's about comfort, culture, and sometimes our most excellent companion after a demanding day. But as we journey through menopause, our relationship with food becomes even more vital. Suddenly, your mood might change significantly depending on your consumption, which is perfectly normal. Knowing that the correct diet can help with everything from controlling hot flashes to preserving bone mass and sustaining energy levels is empowering.

The Function Of Diet In Menopause: How Your Food Affects Your Emotions.

Understanding the whirlpool of symptoms menopause can send your way is the first step to taking control. It's easy to grab comfort foods or skip meals altogether, but the truth is that your body is changing significantly and needs the correct type of nutrition to keep everything working as it should. This knowledge empowers you to make the right choices for your health and well-being.

Reasons It Matters.

During menopause, your metabolism slows down, and your body loses some capacity to absorb certain nutrients. This means you might not get the nutrients you need to feel your best even if you eat the same way you always did. It's important to understand that the hormonal changes associated with menopause can significantly affect your appetite, energy level, and mood; this is a normal part of the process. So, knowing what you place on your plate is even more crucial.

Like many, I never paid much attention to nutrition outside the conventional 'eat your veggies' slogan before menopause. But once I started feeling tired and gaining weight, I knew my regular eating patterns weren't working anymore. Finding the right diet was daunting, but it was a relief to discover that simple adjustments, like eating more nutrient-dense foods and less quick-fix foods, could make a significant difference. This discovery brought hope and encouragement, knowing I could make a positive change.

Key Nutrients For Menopausal Health.

Some nutrients become especially important for your health as you navigate through menopause. These foods assist your body through its changes and help control symptoms.

Calcium and vitamin D: The Bone Guardians.

Menopause highlights the importance of bone health. With the decrease in estrogen levels, the risk of osteoporosis, a condition characterized by brittle bones, becomes a significant and urgent concern. This underscores the crucial role of calcium and vitamin D in your diet. Calcium is essential for the growth and maintenance of strong bones, while vitamin D aids in the absorption of calcium, thereby preventing osteoporosis.

Magnesium: The Agent of Stability for Mood Disorders.

When it comes to menopause, magnesium is quite a Rockstar. It affects everything from emotional control to muscular ability. Low magnesium levels have been related to more symptoms of sadness and anxiety; hence, ensuring enough of this mineral will help in maintaining an even balance of your mood.

Foods Rich In Omega-3 Fatty Acids: The Heart Helpers.

Omega-3 fatty acids, which abound in foods including fish, flaxseeds, and walnuts, become especially crucial given the higher risk of heart disease during post-menopause. They maintain your heart's health, regulate blood pressure, and aid in easing inflammation.

My journey towards better bone health was kickstarted by a crucial discussion about bone density with my doctor. The task of ensuring adequate calcium, vitamin D, and magnesium intake without a major overhaul of my diet seemed daunting at first. However, I soon realized that small changes could make a big difference. It was a journey of discovery and learning, understanding how these nutrients affect bone health. For instance, incorporating a handful of almonds into my morning routine or spending more time outdoors soaking up some vitamin D has proven to be beneficial.

Plant-Based Estrogen: Phytoestrogens and Their Effects.

Phytoestrogens, these naturally occurring molecules found in plants, are a reassuring alternative to hormone treatment. While they can't replace it, they can certainly assist in reducing some menopausal symptoms.

What Are Phytoestrogens?

Beans, flaxseeds, and soy are just a few examples of the diverse range of foods that are high in phytoestrogens. Their modest estrogen-like action comes from binding to estrogen receptors in the body. Including these foods in your diet can help in situations where your body's estrogen levels are dropping throughout menopause.

The Benefits.

Including phytoestrogens in your diet enhances bone health, lessens the severity of hot flashes, and even strengthens heart function. Because the effects vary for everyone, you may have to try several foods to find what works for you.

Like many, I was initially skeptical about phytoestrogens. I couldn't believe that a small amount of soy could make any difference. However, after a few weeks of increasing my flaxseeds and soy milk intake, I noticed a significant reduction in the intensity of my hot flashes. It wasn't a miracle cure, but it was enough of a difference to make me a believer in the power of phytoestrogens.

Foods To Embrace: Building A Menopause-Friendly Diet.

What should you eat to feel best throughout menopause? The good news is that focusing on whole, nutrient-dense meals that assist your body through this transition can help you avoid a complex diet plan. This type of diet has been shown to reduce hot flashes, improve mood, and support overall health during menopause.

Your Nutrient Powerhouses: Fruits and Vegetables.

Your diet should focus on fruits and vegetables. They are not just food; they are your allies, packed with vitamins, minerals, and antioxidants that support everything from your immune system to your skin. Their great fiber count also keeps you feeling full and aids with digestion.

Lean Proteins: The Construction Blocks.

Protein is a key player in preserving muscle mass, especially as we age. Lean proteins like chicken, turkey, tofu, and fish are the perfect solution, providing the necessary building blocks without unnecessary fat. With these lean proteins, you can be confident in your physical health.

Whole Grains: The Energy Conservers.

Whole grains, such as brown rice, quinoa, and oats, are high in nutrients and fibre. They keep your digestive system running smoothly, assist in the control of blood sugar levels, and offer consistent energy. This is because they are complex carbohydrates, which are digested more slowly, providing a steady release of energy throughout the day.

Embracing a menopause-friendly diet was a revelation for me. By simply incorporating more fruits like berries, vegetables like kale, and healthy grains like quinoa into my meals, I experienced a significant shift. I felt more energized, my mood was more stable, and I was less sluggish than before. This transformation is within your reach, too.

Foods To Avoid: Those That Could Make Conditions Worse.

By steering clear of these foods, you can significantly reduce the severity of your menopausal symptoms.

While it's true that many foods can ease menopausal symptoms, it's equally important to recognize that avoiding certain foods can bring relief. This knowledge can fill you with hope and optimism for a more comfortable menopausal experience.

Processed Foods: The Energy Zappers.

Many times, heavy in sugar, salt, and bad fats, processed meals can aggravate menopausal symptoms like weight gain, bloating, and mood swings. They also provide little in terms of nutrients, which makes you feel sluggish and unsatisfied.

Caffeine And Alcohol: The Hot Flash Triggers.

Two things you most definitely do not want more of during menopause are caffeine and alcohol. Caffeine and alcohol can cause hot flashes and disturb your sleep. Reducing your morning coffee or evening glass of wine intake can reduce the frequency and severity of your hot flashes and improve the quality of your sleep.

Sugary Treats: The Mood Swings.

Although it's easy to grab sweets when you're feeling low, sugar can cause your blood sugar levels to surge and plummet, which causes mood swings and tiredness. These goodies are best enjoyed in moderation, meaning you can occasionally have a small piece of dark chocolate or a single cookie, but not as a regular part of your diet.

I used to be a coffee addict, but I decided to cut back when I realized my hot flashes were worse on days when I drank a lot of caffeine. It was difficult; I missed that morning surge of energy, but with time, I found my symptoms were less severe. The slight cost paid for a great benefit. Now, I feel more energetic, and my hot flashes are under control.

Hydration: Drinking Your Way To Improved Wellness.

While the concept of drinking enough water might seem simple, it's a powerful tool, especially during menopause. Ensuring you drink enough water is vital, as dehydration can aggravate symptoms, including hot flashes, headaches, and dry skin. It's a straightforward step that can make a significant difference in your wellness.

Why Hydration Matters During Menopause.

Water preserves your skin moisturized, allows your body temperature to be regulated, and promotes digestion. Maintaining hydration can assist your body through menopause and relieve symptoms like dry skin and tiredness.

Your objective should be to drink at least eight glasses of water daily. But you should pay attention to your body, especially in a hot or busy environment. In such circumstances, your body may need more water. Additionally, herbal teas and meals high in water content, such as fruits and vegetables, help you stay hydrated.

I never considered how much water I was drinking, but after learning about the advantages of staying hydrated, I deliberately tried to drink more all day. My skin was healthier, my energy was higher, and my heat flashes were less severe. Although it's one of the most straightforward adjustments you may make, its effects could be significant.

Vitamins And Their Function: Negotiating The Supplement Aisle.

Understanding the role of supplements in managing menopausal symptoms can be empowering. While food is usually the best source of nutrients, several supplements can support your health throughout menopause and assist in covering for deficiencies. This knowledge puts you in the driver's seat of your health journey.

Get Sufficient Vitamins D and calcium.

Should your diet fail to provide sufficient calcium and vitamin D, supplements can help you meet your needs. These methods are crucial for maintaining bone health and reducing the risk of osteoporosis.

Magnesium Supplements.

Magnesium supplements support sleep, mood control, muscular cramping, and other aspects. If your diet is insufficient, a supplement might be a beneficial addition to your routine.

Omega-3 Fatty Acids.

If you dislike fish or other sources of omega-3s, a supplement can help lower inflammation and maintain heart function.

At first, navigating the supplement shelves was a little daunting — there are so many choices, and knowing the exact supplement I need isn't easy. However, speaking with my doctor and emphasizing the fundamentals — calcium, vitamin D, and magnesium — was beneficial. Although it was just a tiny addition to my daily schedule, it changed my general well-being and energy level. While they are not panacea, supplements can be a helpful tool when used sensibly, providing reassurance and confidence in their effectiveness.

Meal Planning And Recipes: Practical Advice For Eating Well.

Understanding the beneficial foods and those to avoid is just the beginning. The key to a successful menopause-friendly diet is meal planning. It not only ensures you get the necessary nutrition but also saves time and keeps you on track with your health goals.

The Fundamentals of Meal Planning.

Meal planning may sound daunting, but it's actually quite simple. Start by choosing recipes that you enjoy and that include menopause-friendly foods. Then, make a shopping list to ensure you have all the necessary ingredients. Finally, schedule your meals around these dishes. By doing this, you can avoid the stress of preparing dinner after a long day.

Menopause-Friendly Food List.

With a plethora of ideas and comprehensive recipes to guide your everyday meals, let's explore what a menopause-friendly diet might include. The goal is to offer a variety of balanced, nutrient-dense meals that promote health and well-being throughout this transition, leaving you feeling excited and inspired about your meal choices.

Breakfast Menu Options.

1. Flaxseed And Blueberry Oatmeal:

Ingredients:

- Half a cup of rolled oats.
- A single cup of almond milk or any alternative plant-based milk.
- One tablespoon ground flaxseed.

- Half of a cup of blueberries, fresh or frozen.
- One tablespoon chopped walnuts.
- Honey or maple syrup, one teaspoon (if desired).
- A pinch of cinnamon

Preparations:

1. Combine the almond milk and rolled oats in a small pot. Heat over medium flame, stir occasionally and cook until the oats become soft and creamy (approximately 5-7 minutes).
2. Stir in the flaxseeds, cinnamon, and blueberries. Continue cooking for a further minute or until the blueberries reach a warm temperature.
3. Transfer to a bowl, top with chopped walnuts, and drizzle with honey or maple syrup if desired.

Why It's Menopause-Friendly:

This meal is not only high in omega-3 fatty acids from flaxseeds, blueberries, and antioxidants, but they are also easy to prepare and incorporate into your daily routine. Walnuts provide suitable lipids for heart health, and plant-based milk supplies calcium, making it a convenient and menopause-friendly choice.

2. Greek Yoghurt Garnished With a Combination Of Berries, Almonds, And Flaxseeds:

Ingredients:

- One cup of Greek yogurt (unsweetened).
- One tablespoon of ground flaxseeds.
- One-fourth cup of mixed berries (strawberries, raspberries, or blueberries).
- One teaspoon of almonds or walnuts, chopped.
- One teaspoon of honey or agave syrup (optional).

Preparations:

1. Spoon the Greek yoghurt into an empty bowl.
2. Sprinkle the flaxseeds and chopped nuts over the top.
3. Add the mixed berries and drizzle with honey or agave syrup if you like a touch of sweetness.

Why It's Menopause-Friendly:

This meal is a rich source of calcium and protein, two nutrients essential for menopause. The phytoestrogens and omega-3 fatty acids in flaxseeds help control hot flashes and other symptoms, while the antioxidants in berries support general health. The variety of nutrients in this meal will help you feel reassured about your overall health during menopause.

3. Avocado and Egg Toast:

Ingredients:

- A slice of whole grain or rye bread.
- Half of a ripe avocado.
- One egg (boiled, poached, or scrambled).
- A squeeze of lemon juice.
- Salt and pepper to taste.
- A pinch of red pepper flakes (optional).

Preparations:

1. Toast the bread until it reaches the crispiness you prefer.

2. As the bread is toasted, use a fork to crush the avocado in a small bowl with a bit of lemon juice, salt, and pepper.

3. Apply the mashed avocado onto the toast.

4. Top with the egg and sprinkle with red pepper flakes if you like a bit of heat.

Why It's Menopause-Friendly:

Avocados are rich in healthy fats, which help support hormone balance and skin health. Eggs provide high-quality protein and essential vitamins like B12, which can help with energy levels. And then there's whole grain bread, a key player in your diet. It offers a good amount of fiber and complex carbs, which keep you full and satisfied, making it an essential part of managing menopause symptoms.

Lunch Menu Options.

1. Grilled Salmon Salad with Avocado and Spinach:

Ingredients:

- One salmon fillet (about 4-6 ounces)
- Two cups of fresh spinach
- Half of sliced avocado
- One-quarter cup of cherry tomatoes, halved
- One-quarter of a cup of cucumber, sliced
- Two tablespoons red onion, thinly sliced
- One tablespoon olive oil
- One tablespoon lemon juice
- Use salt and pepper to season the food according to your liking.

Preparations:

1. Season the salmon fillet with salt and pepper and grill it over medium heat for 4-5 minutes per side until fully cooked.
2. Combine the spinach, avocado, cherry tomatoes, cucumber, and red onion in a large bowl.
3. Mix the olive oil and lemon juice in a small bowl. Pour the oil over the salad, then toss to coat it.
4. Top the salad with grilled salmon and enjoy.

Why It's Menopause-Friendly:

Salmon is high in omega-3 fatty acids, which help reduce inflammation and improve heart health. Tomatoes and cucumbers add water and fibre, while avocado and spinach supply folate, vitamin K, and healthy fats, promoting overall health during menopause.

2. Quinoa and Black Bean Salad.

Ingredients:

- One cup of cooked quinoa
- Half a cup of black beans, drained and rinsed
- Half red bell pepper, diced
- One-quarter of a cup of fresh or frozen corn kernels.
- One-quarter of a cup of chopped cilantro

- One-quarter of a cup of crumbled feta cheese (optional)
- Two tablespoons of olive oil
- One tablespoon of lime juice
- Half a teaspoon of cumin
- Spice it up with salt and pepper to taste.

Preparations:

1. Combine the cooked quinoa, black beans, red bell pepper, corn, and cilantro in a large bowl.
2. Whisk the olive oil, lime juice, cumin, salt, and pepper in a small bowl.
3. Drizzle the dressing over the salad and mix it well.
4. Add crumbled feta cheese on top if you like.

Why It's Menopause-Friendly:

In addition to being a fantastic source of magnesium necessary for healthy muscles and mood control, quinoa is a complete protein. The vegetables contribute minerals and antioxidants that promote general health, while the black beans give fibre and extra protein.

3. Mediterranean Chickpea Wrap.

Ingredients:

- One whole grain or spinach wrap.
- One-quarter of a cup of canned chickpeas, drained and rinsed.
- One-quarter of a cup of hummus.
- One-quarter of a cup of chopped cucumber.
- A quarter cup of diced tomatoes.
- Two tablespoons crumbled feta cheese.
- Toss in some mixed greens (lettuce, rocket or spinach),
- Drop some lemon juice and olive oil over top,
- Season with salt and pepper to taste.

Preparations:

1. In a bowl, mash the chickpeas slightly with a fork, leaving some whole for texture.
2. Spread the hummus over the wrap.
3. Top with the mashed chickpeas, cucumber, tomatoes, feta cheese, and mixed greens.
4. Drizzle with olive oil and lemon juice, and season with salt and pepper.
5. Roll up the wrap tightly and cut it in half.

Why It's Menopause-Friendly:

Chickpeas, rich in plant-based protein and fiber, are a powerful tool in promoting digestive health and satiety. The fresh vegetables and greens offer essential vitamins and moisture, while the hummus adds healthy fats and a creamy texture.

Dinner Menu Options:

1. Baked Cod with Lemon and Asparagus.

Ingredients:

- Two cod fillets
- One bunch of asparagus, trimmed.
- Two tablespoons of olive oil
- One lemon (zested and juiced).
- Two garlic cloves, minced.
- Add salt and pepper to taste.
- Fresh parsley, chopped (for garnish).

Preparations:

1. Preheat your oven to 400°F (200°C).
2. Place the cod fillets on a baking sheet with parchment paper.

3. In a small bowl, mix the olive oil, lemon zest, lemon juice, and minced garlic.

4. Drizzle the mixture over the cod and asparagus. Season with salt and pepper.

5. Bake for 15-20 minutes until the cod is opaque and flakes easily with a fork and the asparagus is tender.

6. Garnish with fresh parsley before serving.

Why It's Menopause-Friendly:

This meal is a great approach to controlling weight during menopause. Cod is low in calories and a lean protein source, making it a perfect choice for weight management. Asparagus and folate are abundant in Vitamins A, C, and K, promoting heart health and strong bones, giving you the confidence that you are in control of your weight during menopause.

2. Stuffed Bell Peppers with Turkey and Brown Rice.

Ingredients:

- Four large bell peppers (any color).
- One pound ground turkey.
- One cup of cooked brown rice.
- Half onion, diced.
- Two garlic cloves, minced.

- One cup of chopped tomatoes, either fresh or picked from a can.

- One teaspoon dried oregano.

- One teaspoon dried basil.

- Half a cup of shredded mozzarella cheese (optional).

- Add salt and pepper to taste.

Preparations:

1. Preheat your oven to 375°F (190°C).

2. Cut off the bell peppers' tops and remove the seeds and membranes. The peppers should be put in a baking dish.

3. Brown the ground turkey over medium heat in a spacious skillet. Then, add the garlic and onion, cooking them until they become soft.

4. Stir in the cooked brown rice, diced tomatoes, oregano, basil, salt, and pepper. Boil for another five minutes until all the ingredients are thoroughly mixed. This simple step ensures a flavorful and satisfying meal without stress or hassle.

5. Fill the bell peppers with the turkey mixture. If you use cheese, place it on top of each filled pepper.

6. Cover the baking dish with foil and bake for 25-30 minutes until the peppers are tender.

7. Remove the foil and bake for 5 minutes to melt the cheese if using.

Why It's Menopause-Friendly:

Tryptophan, an amino acid that helps control mood and sleep, is abundant in Turkey and is a lean protein source. Brown rice's fiber and complex carbohydrates contribute to blood sugar stabilization. Rich in vitamins A and C, bell peppers promote healthy skin and a robust immune system.

These ingredients are not just delicious; they're a powerhouse of health benefits for menopausal women, providing a strong sense of reassurance and confidence in your dietary choices and empowering you to take control of your health.

3. Lentil and Vegetable Stir-Fry.

Ingredients:

- One cup of cooked lentils (green or brown)
- One cup of bell pepper, sliced
- One cup of zucchini, sliced
- One cup of carrot, julienned
- One cup of cup broccoli florets
- Two tablespoons of olive oil
- Two tablespoons of low-sodium soy sauce.
- One tablespoon of rice vinegar
- One teaspoon of sesame oil
- One garlic clove, minced

- One teaspoon of grated ginger
- Cooked brown rice or quinoa (for serving)
- Sesame seeds and green onions (for garnish)

Preparations:

1. Warm the olive oil in a large frying pan or wok over medium-high heat.
2. Sauté the garlic and ginger for 1-2 minutes until they develop a pleasant aroma.
3. Add the bell pepper, zucchini, carrot, broccoli, and stir-fry for 5-7 minutes until the vegetables are tender but still crisp.
4. Stir in the cooked lentils, soy sauce, rice vinegar, and sesame oil. Cook for two to three minutes until everything is hot.
5. Serve the stir-fry over brown rice or quinoa, and garnish with sesame seeds and sliced green onions.

Why It's Menopause-Friendly:

Lentils are essential for energy levels and digestion and are an exceptional plant-based protein, fiber, and iron source. While sesame oil offers good fats supporting hormone balance, the vivid vegetables provide a range of vitamins and antioxidants, making this stir-fry a perfect choice for menopause management.

Ideas For Snacks:

1. Apple Slices with Almond Butter.

Ingredients:

• One apple, sliced.

• Two tablespoons of almond butter.

Preparations:

1. Core the apple and slice it into wedges.
2. Serve the apple slices with almond butter for dipping.

Why It's Menopause-Friendly:

While almond butter supplies good fats and protein that keep you full and satisfied between meals, apples are high in fiber and vitamin C.

2. Edamame with Sea Salt.

Ingredients:

• One cup of shelled edamame (fresh or frozen).

• A pinch of sea salt.

Preparations:

1. Prepare the edamame by steaming it as directed on the package.

2. Sprinkle with sea salt and enjoy warm or chilled.

Why It's Menopause-Friendly:

Edamame is a fantastic source of phytoestrogens and plant-based proteins, which can help control menopausal symptoms, including hot flashes. It also provides all the nutrients and fiber you need, making it an excellent choice for menopause management.

3. Chia Pudding with Berries.

Ingredients:

- Three tablespoons of chia seeds.

- One teaspoon of honey or maple syrup.

- A cup of almond milk (or a different organic milk).

- Half a cup of mixed berries (strawberries, blueberries, or raspberries).

Preparations:

1. Mix the chia seeds with almond milk and honey or maple syrup in a bowl or jar.

2. Stir well to combine and refrigerate for at least 2 hours, or overnight, until the mixture thickens.

3. Top with fresh berries before serving.

Why It's Menopause-Friendly:

Chia seeds are filling and nutrient-rich, packed with omega-3 fatty acids, fiber, and protein. Berries, on the other hand, are full of vitamins and taste great, making this pudding a perfect choice for managing menopause and ensuring you're getting the health benefits you need.

Dessert Menu Options.

1. Dark Chocolate and Nut Bark

Ingredients:

- One cup of dark chocolate chips (70% cocoa or higher).
- One-quarter cup of almonds, chopped.
- One-quarter cup of walnuts, chopped.
- A pinch of sea salt.

Instructions:

1. Melt the dark chocolate chips in a microwave-safe bowl, heating in 30-second intervals and stirring until smooth.

2. Spread the melted chocolate onto a parchment-lined baking sheet in a thin layer.

3. Sprinkle the chopped nuts and sea salt over the chocolate.

4. Refrigerate until the chocolate is firm, for about 30 minutes.

5. Break into pieces and enjoy.

Why It's Menopause-Friendly:

Dark chocolate, rich in antioxidants, is a reassuring choice for supporting heart health and mood. The addition of nuts, with their healthy fats, protein, and fiber, makes this a balanced and satisfying treat, instilling confidence in its health benefits for a menopause-friendly diet.

2. Baked Apples with Cinnamon and Walnuts.

Ingredients:

- Four apples, cored.

- One-quarter cup of walnuts, chopped.

- Two tablespoons of raisins.

- One tablespoon of honey or maple syrup.

- One teaspoon of ground cinnamon.

<u>Instructions:</u>

1. Preheat your oven to 350°F (175°C).

2. Place the cored apples in a baking dish.

3. In a small bowl, mix the chopped walnuts, raisins, honey or maple syrup, and cinnamon.

4. Stuff the mixture into the center of each apple.

5. Bake for 25-30 minutes until the apples are tender.

6. Serve warm, optionally, with a dollop of Greek yogurt or a scoop of vanilla ice cream.

Why It's Menopause-Friendly:

Baked apples are a tasty and satisfying treat high in fiber and antioxidants. While cinnamon could help control blood sugar levels, adding walnuts empowers you with healthy fats and protein, putting you in control of your health during menopause.

Wrapping up this section.

Eating well during menopause is about nourishing your body with foods that support your life transition needs. With these meal options and recipes, you can create a diet that not only helps manage menopausal symptoms but also keeps you feeling energized and satisfied. Whether you're a seasoned cook or just starting, these recipes are designed to be easy, delicious, and full of the nutrients you need to thrive in this new life phase. So, grab your apron, head to the kitchen, and savor the process of making meals as enjoyable as they are good for you!

Cooking wasn't always my forte, but I discovered a new passion when I started experimenting with delicious menopause-friendly foods. It became a delightful self-care journey, and I found joy in the process. Moreover, I realized that I was empowering myself by providing my body with the necessary nutrients during this period.

Managing menopause relies on nutrition, so finding the right approach may help you feel your best and reduce symptoms. Remember, it's about discovering what works for you and making small, long-term changes to improve your health and well-being; it's not about perfection. Don't forget to enjoy the journey—food is meant to be savored!

Checklist:

- ☐ Review your eating habits to see if any food triggers hot flashes or mood changes.
- ☐ Incorporate calcium-rich foods (dairy, leafy greens, fortified foods) to support bone health.
- ☐ Increase your intake of fiber-rich foods (whole grains, fruits, vegetables).

☐ Drink plenty of water — try to have eight glasses or more each day.

☐ Cut back on caffeine, alcohol, and spicy foods that may trigger symptoms.

Action Plan:

1. **Take Control:** Keep a weekly food diary and note how different foods affect your menopause symptoms. This proactive approach will help you understand your body's unique needs and make informed dietary choices.

2. **Support Your Bones:** Ensure you're eating plenty of foods that support bone health, such as low-fat dairy, almonds, and broccoli. These calcium-rich foods are crucial for maintaining strong bones during menopause.

3. **Boost Fiber Intake:** Incorporate more fiber into your diet by switching to whole grains, adding more fruits and veggies, and considering fiber supplements if necessary.

4. **Nurture Your Body:** Make a conscious effort to drink more water, especially if you have hot flashes or dry skin. This simple act of self-

care can make a significant difference in managing your menopause symptoms.

5. **Limit Triggers:** Identify foods that may exacerbate symptoms (like caffeine or spicy food) and try cutting back or eliminating them for a week to see if it makes a difference.

6. Exercise And Physical Activity During Menopause.

"Don't let menopause slow you down. Keep moving forward." – Unknown

Staying active throughout menopause might seem like finding the proper medication to treat the symptoms of this new phase of life. Exercise is more than simply squeezing into your favorite pair of pants; it is about enhancing your health and well-being.

Let's examine why training is essential during menopause and how to include it, even if cuddling up on the sofa sounds more appealing.

Why Exercise Matters.

Exercise during menopause is a natural energy booster, much like a cup of coffee that kick-starts your day. It revitalizes your body, keeps you energetic, and prepares you for the day.

However, unlike your morning coffee, regular exercise offers a range of long-term health advantages that are especially crucial during menopause, providing you with reassurance and confidence.

Empower Yourself:

Menopause frequently causes weight increase, especially around the abdomen. Regular exercise helps you control your weight by increasing your metabolism, which slows with age and burns off excess calories. Maintaining a healthy weight is essential for several reasons, including lowering your risk of heart disease, diabetes, and high blood pressure. By managing your weight through exercise, you control your health and well-being.

Relief From Discomfort:

Exercise helps minimize hot flashes and night sweats. Physical exercise increases your body's capacity to regulate temperature, resulting in fewer unexpected sweaty periods. This relief from discomfort can significantly improve your quality of life during menopause.

Uplift Your Spirits:

Menopause can cause emotional fluctuations. Fortunately, exercise has a profound mood-enhancing effect. Endorphins, your body's natural feel-good chemicals, are released during physical exercise and can help reduce anxiety and despair. Plus, finishing a workout gives you a sense of success, which enhances your confidence and uplifts your spirits.

Enhancing Sleep:

For people with insomnia, regular exercise might help to enhance the quality of sleep. Physical exercise can help you fall asleep sooner and have a deeper, more peaceful sleep, which is critical when menopause affects your usual sleep habits.

Supporting Bone And Heart Health:

Low estrogen levels increase osteoporosis and heart disease risk. Weight-bearing workouts such as walking, running, and strength training can help preserve bone density by putting stress on the bones and stimulating bone growth. Cardiovascular activities promote heart health by improving circulation and reducing the risk of heart disease.

Types Of Exercise: Strength Training, Cardio, Flexibility, And Balance.

Embracing a diverse range of activities that cater to different health needs can inject excitement and motivation into your fitness journey, helping you maximize the benefits of your workouts.

Strength Training:

Strength exercise, also known as resistance training, promotes muscular growth and maintains bone density, which might decrease after menopause. Lifting weights, utilizing resistance bands, or performing bodyweight exercises like squats and push-ups all help to maintain healthy muscles and bones. The more muscle you have, the greater your resting metabolic rate, which helps with weight management.

Remember, you don't have to start with heavy weights. Begin with what feels comfortable and gradually increase. I started with soup cans and then worked towards dumbbells. Trust me, even modest steps can lead to significant progress, so don't be discouraged!

Cardio:

Cardiovascular exercise gets your heart pumping and blood flowing, which is essential for heart health. Activities like walking, jogging, cycling, swimming, or even dancing can help improve cardiovascular endurance, reduce stress, and burn calories.

I never thought I'd be the person who enjoys running, but after starting a "Special Fitness" program, I found it was a great way to clear my mind and feel more energetic. Plus, there's something satisfying about outpacing a teenager on the treadmill next to you. Sharing my journey is not just about me, but about inspiring you to find your own fitness path.

Flexibility And Balance:

Flexibility and balance exercises are critical for preserving mobility and minimizing injuries as we age. Yoga, Pilates, and regular stretching help keep your muscles supple and enhance your balance, lowering your chance of falling.

Developing A Workout Plan: Tailoring Exercises To Your Needs.

Designing an exercise plan during menopause is not about pushing yourself to the limit; it's about creating a regimen that adapts to your body and lifestyle, putting you in the driver's seat of your fitness journey.

Here's how to create a balanced fitness program:

1. **Begin Slowly:** If you're new to exercising or are getting back into it, start with 10-15 minutes each day and gradually increase the duration and intensity as your stamina improves.

2. **Mix It Up:** Variety is important, and it's exciting. Combining strength training, cardio, flexibility, and balance exercises make

your regimen enjoyable and keeps you engaged in all aspects of your health.

3. **Listen To Your Body:** Menopause is unpredictable. Some days, you may feel exhausted or in pain, while others you may not. It's important to pay attention to your body's signals during workouts and adjust the intensity accordingly. Remember, relaxation days are not just important; they show you care for your body's needs!

4. **Make It Enjoyable:** Exercise does not have to be a hassle. Find activities you enjoy, such as dancing, hiking, or swimming, and include them in your schedule.

Bone Health: Strengthening And Protecting Your Bones.

Menopause raises the risk of osteoporosis owing to decreasing estrogen levels; thus, maintaining bone health is crucial.

Weight-Bearing Exercises:

Weight-bearing workouts such as walking, running, and stair climbing promote bone density by working against gravity. Stronger bones may be developed even from small deeds like brushing your teeth while standing on one foot.

Regular exercise throughout menopause and a balanced diet can help control symptoms and enhance general health, leaving you strong during this vital period.

Strength Training for Bones:

Strength training is essential for bone health as much as for muscle development. Resistance bands or weightlifting increase bone development and help prevent bone loss.

High-impact Workouts:

Although high-impact workouts (such as running or leaping) might be demanding, they are great for preserving and increasing bone density. If you have never done these exercises, start small — jumping jacks in your living room will be a perfect start.

I recall being afraid of lifting weights because I thought I might injure myself. Starting with modest dumbbells and progressively raising the weight, however, not only developed my muscles but also provided me with mental peace of mind, knowing I was preserving my bones.

Engage In Cardiovascular Exercises For A Healthy Heart.

After menopause, the risk of heart disease rises; thus, maintaining a healthy heart is vital.

Walking

Among the most accessible and potent cardiovascular activities is walking. Try to get thirty minutes five days a week. It's low-impact and gentle on the joints; you can do it anywhere.

Interval Training

Interval training entails alternating between intensive exercise and rest/lower intensity. For example, during a stroll, you may walk quickly for one minute and then at a moderate pace for two minutes. This method of training can enhance cardiovascular fitness faster than steady-state cardio.

Swimming & Cycling:

Swimming and cycling are great for people with joint issues or those seeking low-impact activities. They increase heart rate without taxing the hips or knees.

Exercises For The Pelvic Floor: Building The Foundation.

Menopause can weaken pelvic floor muscles, leading to issues like pelvic organ prolapse or incontinence. Strengthening these muscles is vital. However, seeking guidance from a healthcare professional before embarking on any new exercise routine is crucial, especially if you have pre-existing health conditions.

Kegel Exercises:

Kegels are exercises for the pelvic floor muscles that alternately contract and release. To engage in a Kegel exercise, which involves holding the flow of urination midway, retaining the contraction briefly and then letting go, follow these steps:

1. Find a relaxed position, whether sitting or lying down.
2. Squeeze your pelvic floor muscles as if trying to stop the urine flow.
3. Hold the contraction for 3-5 seconds, then relax for the same amount of time.
4. Repeat this 10-15 times, a few times daily.

Mastering Kegel exercises is a personal triumph that can empower you in ways you never imagined. These exercises, which can be done discreetly while watching TV, are game changers. They are effortless and understated, yet rather powerful, giving you a sense of control over your body.

Yoga For The Pelvic Floor:

Several yoga positions, such as child's and bridge poses, may strengthen the pelvic floor. These postures are excellent additions to your program as they gently, under control, impact the muscles.

Yoga And Mind-Body Practices: Embracing Calm Through Movement.

For menopause, yoga and other mind-body techniques, such as Tai Chi and meditation, are excellent for both physical and psychological wellness.

Yoga For Flexibility And Strength:

Excellent all-around exercise yoga for flexibility and strength enhances balance, flexibility, and strength. While helping you relax, poses such as downward dog, warrior II, and tree pose to stretch and strengthen your muscles.

Breathwork And Meditation:

Tension and anxiety, which are common during menopause, can be managed with breathwork and meditation. Deep breathing and mindfulness meditation help one relax, promoting peace and enhancing sleep quality.

Tai Chi:

Tai chi is a calm, flowing activity that increases mental clarity, flexibility, and balance. It also significantly improves attention and lowers stress.

I fell out of positions more often than I held when I first started yoga. However, I discovered my flow through practice and recognized that yoga is more about mental balance than physical flexibility.

Overcoming Obstacles To Exercise.

It is crucial to stay active even when you don't feel like it. Days will pass when you find yourself not motivated to work out. You might be bored, not in the mood, or exhausted.

Here's how one may get around such obstacles:

1. **Set Small, Achievable Goals:**
    The Key to Overcoming Obstacles. On days when you lack motivation, commit to just ten minutes of exercise. Once you start, you'll often find yourself more invigorated and accomplishing more than you had planned, boosting your motivation and sense of achievement.

2. **Get A Workout Buddy.**
    Exercise with a buddy, enroll in a class or participate in a collective project. Make it social. Having someone to share the experience with helps you be responsible and makes it more fun.

3. **Discover Joy In Movement.**
    Recall that exercise should not be structured. Gardening, dancing around the home, and going on a nature walk are all physical activities. The secret is to keep going in the direction of your happiness.

4. **Make Self-Care A Priority and remember that exercise qualifies as such.** It's about encouraging your body, not about punishing it.

Discover hobbies that provide you with mental as well as physical pleasure.

On days when I genuinely want to avoid working out, I promise myself a reward — like a nice bath or a piece of dark chocolate — afterwards. How inspiring a small treat can be is fantastic!

Finally.

Improving general health and controlling menopausal symptoms is a journey that we're all on, and it starts with exercise and physical activity. Strength training, cardio, flexibility, and balance exercises can help lay a solid foundation for a bright, healthy life.

Keep in mind that the goal is to keep improving and not being perfect. Every movement counts, whether it's yoga, weightlifting, or just a walk; it will help all of us take a step closer to feeling our best during menopause. So, unroll your yoga mat, lace your sneakers, or grab those dumbbells — it's time for all of us to welcome the power of movement!

Checklist:

- ☐ Include two to three times a week of weight training in your workout regimen.
- ☐ Add cardio workouts to boost your heart health and manage weight.
- ☐ Practice balance exercises to reduce the risk of falls and injuries.
- ☐ Include flexibility training like yoga or Pilates to support joint health and reduce stiffness.
- ☐ Try short, regular exercise sessions (10-20 minutes) if full workouts feel overwhelming.

Action Plan:

1. **Strength Training:** Start with light weights or bodyweight exercises to build strength and support bone density.

2. **Cardio Workouts:** Aim for at least 30 minutes of moderate-intensity cardio exercises, like brisk walking or swimming, most days of the week.

3. **Balance and Flexibility:** Enhance your stability and security by incorporating balance exercises, such as standing on one foot, and flexibility exercises, like yoga or stretching routines, into your weekly schedule.

4. **Small, Consistent Efforts:** If full workouts seem daunting, start with 10-minute sessions and gradually build from there.

5. **Exercise Routine:** Empower yourself by creating a flexible weekly exercise plan with strength, cardio, and flexibility exercises tailored to your fitness level. This plan is yours to modify and adjust as you see fit, giving you complete control over your fitness journey.

7. Lifestyle Changes That Will Make A Difference During Menopause.

"Menopause is a natural part of aging, and it's nothing to be ashamed of." – Anonymous

Menopause is a unique journey for each woman, and it's essential to remember that what works for one person may not work for another. Before considering hormone replacement therapy, it's crucial to consult with a healthcare professional to understand the potential risks and benefits. However, making innovative changes to your lifestyle can offer hope and help you navigate menopause more comfortably. Even though these changes won't eliminate all your symptoms immediately, they can significantly improve your daily feelings, motivating you to continue on this path.

Let's examine two of the most critical areas: dealing with stress and getting a good night's sleep.

How To Deal With Stress: Specific Yoga And Meditation Techniques To Stay Calm.

Stress is the lightning that strikes during menopause. It comes out of nowhere, shocking everything and making you feel stressed. Not only is it essential to deal with worry for your mental health, but it can also make many menopausal symptoms worse, such as hot flashes, sleep problems, and mood swings.

Why Managing Stress Is Essential:

During menopause, your body is already adjusting to changing hormone levels. When stress is added to the mix, it's like pouring fuel on a fire. Understanding this can bring relief, as it helps you comprehend why your body reacts the way it does.

Our bodies naturally produce the hormone cortisol when we are under stress. This can further disrupt your already delicate biological balance. If your cortisol levels are too high, you might experience weight gain, especially around your belly region, have trouble sleeping, and worsen your hot flashes. The connection between stress and these symptoms is that high cortisol levels can increase fat storage, disrupt sleep patterns, and trigger hot flashes.

When I had a hot flash during a stressful work meeting, I felt like I would blow up. That's when I knew I had to do something about my worry.

Finding Your Balance In Yoga And Outside Of The Mat.

Yoga isn't just an excellent way to work out; it's also a great way to deal with stress. Moving your body, paying attention to your breath, and being aware are all parts of yoga that help to calm the nervous system and lower cortisol levels.

Stretching isn't enough; you need to make room in your mind and body to breathe and release stress.

- **Good for your body:**
  Yoga makes you more flexible, stronger, and balanced, which is essential as your body adjusts to menopause. Child's pose, downward dog, and savasana (corpse pose) are some poses that can help you relax and loosen up your muscles. You can try mindfulness meditation, where you focus on your breath, a word, or a phrase, and when your mind wanders, you slowly bring it back to this focus.

- **Mental Health Advantages:**

One part of yoga, mindfulness, teaches you to focus on the present moment. By doing so, you may have less anxiety and be better able to deal with stress. Deep breathing and focus during yoga classes can help your brain stay calm even when things around you get crazy.

It took me a while to understand what yoga was all about until I tried it. But after a few classes, I understood that yoga was more about getting my mind out of knots. Doing a few sun salutations every morning has become my favorite way to relieve stress.

What Meditation Is All About.

Meditation is like taking a short trip with your mind. You can relax in bed, on your couch, or even in your car (as long as it's parked, of course). No special tools or specific location is required. Meditation is intended to calm your mind and distract you from the things stressing you out.

- **Mindfulness Meditation:**

In this type of meditation, you focus on your breath, a word, or a phrase, and when your mind wanders, you slowly bring it back to this focus. You should be able to get your thoughts back without judging them when they go astray from your primary focus.

- **Guided Meditation:**

  If sitting still scares you, try guided meditation. On apps like *Headspace* and *Calm*, you can do sessions with a calming voice that walks you through the steps. These sessions are usually about sleep, stress relief, or rest.

My initial perception of meditation was that it involved sitting down idly and doing nothing. Then I tried it and realized it was the most challenging "nothing" I've ever done. But it's also the most rewarding. After a 10-minute session, I feel like I've hit the reset button on my day. For instance, I approached a problematic work meeting with a clearer mind and more patience.

Stay Calm When Going Through Menopausal Storm.

Let's be honest — menopause can push your buttons. But learning how to manage your reactions can help you stay grounded and grow. It's not about never getting stressed; it's about learning how to handle stress in a way that doesn't derail your day (or your sanity).

Breathe Deeply:

Take a deep breath when you feel stress creeping in. Breathe in for four seconds, pause for four seconds, and breathe out for four seconds. This simple yet powerful technique can effectively calm your nervous system, allowing you to respond thoughtfully rather than impulsively.

Create a Stress-Free Zone:

Having a designated 'stress-free zone' in your home is crucial. It could be a cozy corner with a comfortable chair, some plants, and your favorite books. Retreating to this space when you're feeling overwhelmed can be a game-changer, helping you reset and regain your balance.

I've turned my bathroom into a stress-free zone. It has candles, essential oils, and a stash of bath bombs. When the day gets too crazy, I retreat there for a soak and much-needed quiet time.

Sleep Hygiene: Creating A Sleep-Friendly Environment.

Sleep and menopause often don't get along. Night sweats, hot flashes, and a mind that won't quit can turn bedtime into a battleground. But sleep is crucial — without it, everything from your mood to your metabolism takes a hit. Good sleep hygiene is about creating the best possible conditions for restful sleep.

Why Sleep Hygiene Matters:

Sleep is when your body repairs itself, processes the day's events, and resets for tomorrow. During menopause, your body works overtime to adjust to hormonal changes, making sleep even more important. But it's not just about quantity —quality sleep is vital to feeling rested and ready to face the day.

There was a time when I thought I could power through with just a few hours of sleep a night. But after waking up feeling like I'd been hit by a truck one too many times, I knew I had to change my approach to sleep. If you are experiencing a similar challenge, remember that you are not the only one facing it.

Prepare A Place That Is Good For Sleep.

Your bedroom should be a place of peace, not stress. Here are some ways to make it easier to sleep:

- **Cool It Down:** It's a good idea to keep your bedroom comfortable, ideally between 60- and 67-degrees Fahrenheit. Sleeping in a more relaxed room is easier because it prevents sweating at night.

- **Darkness is Important:** Make your room as dark as possible. Exposure to light can inhibit your body's production of melatonin, which controls sleep. If you can't stand bright lights, you might want to try dark shade curtains or an eye mask.

- **Comfortable Bedding:** Buy good sheets and a mattress that supports your body. Cotton and other natural fabrics let air pass through them, which can help you stay cool.

- **Please be quiet:** Even if you don't fully wake up, noise can wake you up. If you live in a loud area, you might want to use earplugs or a white noise machine to block out disturbing sounds.

It's like being in a bat cave in my bedroom, but there are no bats. I can say for sure that it has changed the way I sleep.

Set Up A Bedtime Routine.

Sleep practice is suitable for both kids and adults. It tells your body it's time to relax and prepare for bed.

- **<u>Regular Bedtime:</u>** Every day, even on the weekends, go to bed and wake up at the same time. This helps keep your body's clock in sync, making it easier to fall asleep and wake up naturally.

- **<u>Relax Before Bed:</u>** Take at least 30 minutes before sleeping to "wind down". In this case, you might read, take a warm bath, or do some easy yoga. During this time, stay away from computers because the blue light from phones and tablets can stop your body from making melatonin.

- **<u>Don't Drink Too Much Alcohol or Caffeine</u>**. Both substances could make it challenging to get or stay asleep. Avoid coffee in the afternoon and evening, and drink less alcohol, especially right before bed.

I used to think caffeine couldn't hurt me until I had an espresso at 4 p.m. and was wide awake at midnight, feeling terrible about everything I had done. In the afternoon, I now drink green tea.

How To Get Sleep If You Can't.

There will be nights when you can't fall asleep, no matter how hard you try. Do these things:

- **<u>Get Up:</u>** If you've been in bed for 20 minutes or more without falling asleep, get up and do something calm in a different room. You can read a book, listen to music that makes you feel relaxed, or do deep breathing until you fall asleep.

- **<u>Don't Look At The Clock.</u>** Looking at the clock makes you feel more stressed and makes you worry about how little sleep you're getting. Switch the clock around or hide it to avoid the urge.

- **<u>Use Relaxation Methods.</u>** Guided visualization or gradual muscle relaxation techniques can calm a rushing mind, calm thoughts, and prepare the body for a good night's sleep.

I've found that doing something mindless, like folding clothes, can help me fall asleep on those rare nights when I can't. It's so dull that I want to go back to sleep, but it's better than being stressed out there.

In Conclusion.

Managing stress and creating a sleep-friendly setting are two of the most helpful changes you can make to your lifestyle to make menopause more manageable. Even though these habits won't fix everything, they can help make the journey easier.

Remember that the goal is growth, not perfection. So, every step you take toward feeling your best, like learning to do deep breathing or making your bedroom a sleep haven, is a step in the right direction.

Checklist:

☐ Set a routine for yoga, meditation, or other relaxation techniques.

☐ Create a bedtime routine prioritizes relaxation (dim lights, no screens).

☐ Evaluate your daily habits to identify potential stress triggers.

☐ Look into local or online resources for yoga or meditation classes.

Action Plan:

1. **<u>Establish Stress Management Practices:</u>** Incorporate meditation, yoga, or deep breathing exercises into your daily routine.

2. **<u>Improve Sleep Hygiene:</u>** Create a calming sleep environment by reducing light, screens, and noise before bedtime. Evaluate your daily habits by journaling your activities and emotions to identify potential stress triggers.

3. **<u>Plan Relaxation Time:</u>** Set aside 15-30 minutes daily for self-care activities that calm your mind. This could include reading a book, bathing, or walking in nature.

4. **<u>Experiment With Relaxation Methods:</u>** Foster a sense of curiosity and open-mindedness by trying different stress-relief practices, such

as journaling, aromatherapy, or progressive muscle relaxation, to see what works best for you.

8. Hormone Replacement Therapy (HRT).

"Menopause is not the end, it's a new beginning. Embrace the changes and find strength within." – Anonymous

A lot of different feelings can be stirred up by the subject of Hormone Replacement Therapy (HRT). Some people see it as a lifesaver that helps them get through menopause, while others see it as a scary idea with too many unknowns.

If you're thinking about HRT or want to know what all the fuss is about, this chapter will explain it all for you. It will cover what HRT is, the different types, the risks, and the stories of real women who have used it (or not).

What Does HRT Mean?

To begin, let us look at the basics. One way to ease the signs of menopause is with Hormone Replacement Therapy, which replaces the hormones that your body isn't making enough of on its own. As menopause approaches, there is a decrease in estrogen and progesterone levels. This drop can cause a lot of problems, such as hot flashes, night sweats, mood swings, and tightness in the vaginal area. These hormones are added to HRT to help bring your body back into balance.

How Does HRT Do Its job?

HRT comes in many forms, such as pills, patches, creams, gels, and even vaginal rings. Your doctor may give you Estrogen-only Treatment (ET) or a mix of ET and Progesterone (EPT), depending on your symptoms and health history. If you have undergone a hysterectomy, you might require estrogen only. However, if your uterus is intact, you'll probably need both hormones to reduce the likelihood of developing uterine cancer.

When I heard about HRT for the first time, I thought it would be like a complicated science project with sparks and beakers. But the truth is that HRT is relatively easy to understand. My doctor and I talked about my symptoms and looked at the different choices. I learned that it's more about finding the right fit for your body and way of life.

Why Consider HRT?

Hormone Replacement Therapy (HRT) helps many women with their menopause symptoms. It helps even more if your symptoms are bad, making your life less enjoyable. For example, if you always wake up soaked in sweat or feel like your emotions are all over the place, HRT might give you the balance you need to feel like yourself again.

What Are The Benefits And Drawbacks? - Is This Appropriate For You?

Making the very personal decision to utilize HRT comes with no one-size-fits-all response. Here is a summary of the advantages and drawbacks to enable you to assess your choices.

<u>*The Benefits Are:*</u>

1. **Relief:** For many of the most prevalent menopausal symptoms, HRT is quite successful in either lowering or eradicating them. Many women find great life-changing relief from hot flashes, night sweats, and vaginal dryness.

2. **Bone Health:** Maintaining bone density depends critically on estrogen. HRT can help prevent bone loss, which causes osteoporosis, by augmenting estrogen and lowering your age-related fracture risk.

3. **Heart Health:** Some studies indicate that HRT may lower the risk of heart disease if begun early in menopause, but this advantage decreases if it is started later in life.

4. **Quality of Life:** HRT can drastically improve daily living for women whose menopausal symptoms are severe, therefore enhancing sleep, mood, and general well-being.

I used to joke that my hot flashes were so severe that I could toast marshmallows from my body heat. HRT lowered the temperature so much that I might have to save the s'mores for the campfire!

The Drawbacks:

1. Risks Of Blood Clots And Stroke:

HRT — especially in tablet form — can raise the risk of blood clots and stroke, especially in women over 60 or those with existing risk factors like smoking or obesity.

2. Breast Cancer:

The mixture of estrogen and progesterone in HRT has been related to a modest rise in the risk of breast cancer, particularly with long-term usage. The level of risks involved is determined by what kind of HRT is being administered and how long it will take.

3. Side Effects:

Some women get adverse symptoms, including headaches, breast sensitivity, and bloating. Finding the correct dosage and approach that reduces these side effects might take some time.

4. Solution Not Permanent:

Usually used only temporarily, HRT is not a permanent fix. Some symptoms may recur after you stop taking it, so you should discuss your choice to quit HRT with your doctor.

Having balanced the advantages and drawbacks, I decided to try HRT. Making this decision took time — I researched papers and spoke with my doctor for hours. But after I began, my symptoms improved practically right away. Reversing some of the vitality and equilibrium I had lost to menopause, I felt as though I had been given the keys to a time machine.

Personal Stories: Actual Decisions, Real Women.

Every woman's HRT experience is different. Hence, hearing from others who have been through it may be beneficial. These are some personal stories that could resonate with you:

Marilyn's Path to Relief.

Menopause arrived for Marilyn like a freight train in the early 50s. She hardly slept, and the hot flashes persisted nonstop. She eventually discussed HRT with her doctor after trying every natural therapy she could come across — herbs, acupuncture, you name it. Concerned about the hazards, Marilyn hesitated but realized her quality of life came first.

She said she felt a sense of self-identity for the first time in weeks. *"I regained my energy; the hot flashes stopped; I had a restful night's sleep. Hormone replacement therapy transformed my life."*

The Balancing Act of Kimberly.

Given her family history of breast cancer, Kimberly was somewhat wary of thinking about HRT. She chose to try a low-dose estrogen patch after much study and doctor discussions. She felt uneasy but understood that she could no longer endure these symptoms. She recalled: *"I believe I am taking the proper steps for my health, and the patch has worked wonders for my mood swings and night sweats. All of it is about striking equilibrium."*

Annette's Natural Approach.

Annette decided to forego HRT altogether. She said, *"I wanted to see if lifestyle modifications would help me control my symptoms."* Annette concentrated on diet, exercise, and stress management; although initially difficult, she finally developed a schedule that suited her. Though it's not easy, she said she feels powerful knowing she is managing menopause on her terms. *"All women have the right to determine what is most suitable for themselves."*

Different Types of HRT Treatment.

There are various kinds to pick from, and HRT is not a one-size-fits-all therapy. The different options are as follow:

1. Pills:

Pills are one of the most often used types of HRT, they are easy to take and generally available. But they run more danger of blood clots than other kinds of HRT, especially in older women.

2. Patches:

Wearing HRT patches on the skin lets hormones into the bloodstream. They are an excellent alternative if you wish to skip the digestive tract and have a reduced risk of blood clots than pills.

3. Creams and Gels:

When applied to the skin, topical creams and gels are absorbed into the blood circulation. If you have vaginal dryness, their more targeted approach might help.

4. Vaginal Rings:

These low-dose estrogen-releasing flexible rings are placed into the vagina. Vaginal rings mainly help with vaginal dryness and pain without compromising the overall body.

5. Injections:

Hormone injections immediately pump a dosage into the blood circulation and are less frequent but still accessible. They are usually utilized in specific cases and are under careful medical supervision.

I began with an HRT patch as I wanted a consistent hormone release, free of the peaks and valleys associated with pills. Finding the ideal dosage required trial and error, but my body seemed back on an even keel once I did. Night sweats are done, and at last, I felt I could face the day free from the fog of menopause hovering over me.

The Risks and Controversies: Separating Fact from Fiction.

HRT has been the subject of much discussion and study in recent years. Understanding the risks and controversies will enable you to make wiser decisions.

The Risks Are:

1. **Breast Cancer:** The most crucial issue about HRT is the possible rise in breast cancer risk, particularly with long-term mixture of estrogen and progesterone treatment. The risk is usually minor, but it rises with the length of HRT treatment.

2. **Heart Disease and Stroke:** Particularly in women starting HRT later in life, HRT can raise the risk of heart disease and stroke. For some women, though, starting HRT early at the start of menopause may reduce heart disease risk.

3. **Blood Clots:** Estrogen pills raise the likelihood of blood clots, which can cause pulmonary embolism or Deep Vein Thrombosis (DVT). Lower risk is linked to non-oral formulations of HRT, including gels and patches.

The Controversies Are:

1. The Women's Health Initiative (WHI) Study:

Linking HRT to a higher risk of breast cancer, heart disease, and stroke, the 2002 Women's Health Initiative (WHI) research generated great public outcry. Further studies, particularly for younger women or those beginning HRT early in menopause, have indicated, however, that the hazards might not be as significant as first believed.

2. Bioidentical Hormones:

Promoted as a "natural" replacement for conventional HRT, bioidentical hormones, usually manufactured in pharmacies, are chemically identical to the hormones generated by the human body. However, bioidentical hormones are not controlled in the same manner as traditional HRT, and little data indicates they are either safer or more effective.

Steering through the world of HRT is like attempting to find your way through a maze using a constantly changing map. The good news is, though, there is a way out — and it's different for each person.

Separating Fact from Fiction:

A lot of information — and false information — is available regarding HRT that could make the decision-making process seem daunting. Here's how you sort through the clutter and concentrate on what counts:

1. Understand The Research.

Review current research and discuss the most recent findings with your physician. Since the early 2000s, research on HRT has changed drastically; more recent studies provide a more understanding of the dangers and benefits. For instance, commencing HRT early at the start of menopause seems to pose less risk than commencing it later in life.

2. Think About Your Risk Factors.

Whether HRT is appropriate for you depends largely on your unique health profile. Your age, family history, personal medical history, and degree of symptoms will affect your choice.

3. Clarify Your Choices:

Menopause symptoms can be controlled other than with HRT. Alternative therapy, lifestyle modifications, and non-hormonal treatments abound and could potentially help. Talk to your doctor about all your choices so you may decide with knowledge.

4. It Is All About Your Instincts.

The choice to employ HRT is ultimately yours. If it does not seem right or the dangers make you uneasy, you can look at alternative options. On the other hand, don't let fear or false information stop you if HRT looks like the best method you can use to control your symptoms. You are familiar with your body and what works best for it.

When I started looking into HRT, I thought I was drowning in a sea of contradicting information. Every piece expressed something different, and I fretted about choosing the incorrect path. After seeing my doctor and weighing my symptoms, though, I decided to try HRT. Though it wasn't a simple choice, once I started, I found that the advantages were much more than the drawbacks. These days, I believe in doing what feels best for your body — if that is, HRT, a modified lifestyle, or both together.

In conclusion:

Though it's not without complexity, hormone replacement therapy can be an excellent tool for controlling menopausal symptoms. The secret is to stay educated, work closely with your doctor, and decide based on your comfort level and medical requirements. Remember, the exact approach that fits you will help you negotiate menopause; there is no "one right way."

Take a deep breath if the choices and information overwhelm you. Help is available at every turn; you are not journeying this road alone. Whether you decide on HRT or another method, the aim is to feel well in your body and lead your best life during menopause and beyond.

Checklist:

- ☐ Research the different forms of HRT (patches, creams, pills).
- ☐ Write down any concerns or questions you have about HRT to discuss with your doctor.
- ☐ Understand the risks and benefits associated with HRT.
- ☐ Review your personal and family medical history for any conditions that may impact your decision about HRT.

Action Plan:

1. **Gather Information:** Research the different types of HRT and how they work.

2. **Please consult a Professional:** It's essential to book an appointment with your doctor to discuss whether HRT is the right choice for you. Their expert advice will be invaluable in your decision-making process.

3. **Evaluate Risks:** Write down any personal concerns about HRT (e.g., side effects, family history of certain diseases) and ask your doctor about them. This step is crucial in addressing any concerns you may have about HRT.

4. **Weigh the Pros and Cons:** By listing HRT's potential benefits and drawbacks, you can take control of your decision-making process and feel empowered in your choice.

9. Non-Hormonal Treatments.

"Menopause is proof that you can rise, no matter what life throws your way. You've survived, thrived, and now it's time to live fully." — Unknown

Non-hormonal treatments are a valuable option, offering a range of benefits from addressing health concerns to aligning with personal preferences. By exploring these options, you can effectively manage menopausal symptoms without introducing additional hormones into your body.

Drugs And Supplements: Navigating The Pharmacy Aisle.

With shelves stuffed with drugs and supplements all promising to fix your menopausal problems, the pharmacy aisles might seem like a maze. Here, we provide a list of possible challenges and offer guidance on worthwhile choices, supporting your journey to find the right treatment and reducing the overwhelming feeling of choice.

Prescription Drugs:

- **Antidepressants (SSRIs and SNRIs):** Though you are not depressed, certain antidepressants might surprisingly help to lower mood swings and hot flashes. By influencing the neurotransmitters in the brain, drugs such as fluoxetine (Prozac) and venlafaxine (Effexor) assist in regulating mood and lessen the frequency of hot flashes.

- **Gabapentin:** Initially used for epilepsy, gabapentin helps lower hot flashes —especially those that strike at night. If you're seeking a non-hormonal substitute and your symptoms are severe, it can be an excellent choice.

- **Clonidine:** Usually used to treat high blood pressure, clonidine has also been demonstrated to lower hot flash frequency and degree. It influences the blood vessels, therefore controlling the body's temperature.

When my hot flashes first began, I was prepared to endure them, believing no medication could help. But after a tough week of restless nights, I spoke with my doctor. Surprisingly, she suggested an SSRI, which made a significant difference. My mood stabilized, and the hot flashes became more manageable. It wasn't the path I had envisioned, but I'm optimistic that you, too, can find relief in non-hormonal treatments.

Over-the-Counter Supplements:

Before incorporating any over-the-counter treatments into your regimen, it's crucial to consult your doctor. This decision ensures that the treatment is safe and suitable for your specific needs, providing safety and reassurance in your treatment decisions. It's also important to have regular check-ups with your doctor while using these supplements to monitor their effectiveness and any potential side effects.

- **Black Cohosh:** This herb, with its centuries-old history in treating menopausal symptoms, particularly hot flashes and night sweats, is generally considered safe for short-term use. While the scientific evidence is mixed, many women swear by it. However, it's always best to talk to your doctor before adding it to your regimen for that extra layer of reassurance and confidence.

- **Soy Isoflavones:** Isoflavones in soybeans are plant-based estrogens (phytoestrogens) that may offer a promising solution to lower hot flashes. Some trials, particularly for women with moderate symptoms, reveal minor advantages, instilling hope for effective symptom management.

- **Red Clover:** Often recommended as a natural cure for hot flashes and other menopausal symptoms, red clover is another phytoestrogen source. Although the data is conflicting, attempting it under a doctor's direction is usually safe, providing a sense of reassurance and confidence in your choices.

- **Evening Primrose Oil:** Rich in gamma-linolenic acid (GLA), it is supposed to help with hot flashes and breast discomfort. Although the research is scant, some women find it useful, encouraging you to explore its potential benefits.

- **Vitamin E:** Certain research indicates that vitamin E might help lessen the severity of heat flashes. It's also a potent antioxidant; hence, regardless of menopause, it's a beneficial addition to your diet.

Searching the supplement shelves is like trying to choose a new shade of lipstick — there are many choices, and you're not quite sure whether it will work until you get home and test it. With supplements, you won't have to worry about matching your clothing!

Vaginal Moisturizers And Lubricants: Preserving Comfort.

One of those menopausal symptoms that nobody discusses is vaginal dryness, although it's frequent and may significantly affect your comfort and intimacy. Fortunately, a wide range of items are available, giving you the power to choose what's best for you.

Lubricants.

Enhance your intimacy with the transformative power of a good lubricant. Go for water-based ones like **Astroglide** for better comfort and longer-lasting effects or silicone-based ones like **Pjur.** If you're prone to yeast infections, steer clear of glycerin products, as they could worsen your condition.

Vaginal Moisturizers.

Unlike lubricants, which are used during sexual activity, vaginal moisturizers are designed for consistent daily use to maintain vaginal tissue hydration. They help preserve vaginal wall flexibility and moisture. Popular choices include K-Y Liquibeads and Replens, which are easy to use and can help reduce dryness and irritation over time.

When I first went for a vaginal moisturizer, I felt a little embarrassed — like I was confessing defeat to menopause. Still, after a few weeks of use, I saw that it was among my wise choices. The agony disappeared, and I felt like myself once again. Ladies, it's not shameful to keep things cozy!

Acupuncture, Aromatherapy, And Other Mind-Body Techniques.

For women navigating the challenges of menopause, the relief and comfort that mind-body practices can bring are as significant as their physical benefits. These techniques can effectively reduce stress, improve mood, and even alleviate physical symptoms, offering a beacon of hope in the midst of change.

Acupuncture:

This age-old Chinese technique of acupuncture, with its focus on balancing energy flow (Qi), offers a natural, drug-free approach to menopause management. Its proven benefits in improving sleep and mood and reducing hot flashes empower you to take control of your symptoms confidently.

My journey with acupuncture was one of transformation. Initially skeptical, I found that the needles, far from being a discomfort, were a gateway to relaxation and relief. The reduction in the intensity of my hot flashes was a tangible sign of the power of these techniques, inspiring me to continue my holistic approach to menopause management.

Aromatherapy:

Several essential oils—including lavender, peppermint, and clary sage—can help ease menopausal symptoms by encouraging relaxation, enhancing sleep, and regulating hormones. These oils can be added to a warm bath or diffuser or topically diluted with a carrier oil.

Meditation And Mindfulness:

Practicing mindfulness and meditation can help you stay grounded and manage the emotional ups and downs of menopause. Techniques like deep breathing, guided imagery, and progressive muscle relaxation can also reduce stress and improve sleep.

Yoga And Tai Chi:

These mind-body practices combine physical movement with mindfulness, helping to reduce stress, improve flexibility, and enhance overall well-being. Yoga, in particular, can be beneficial for reducing hot flashes and improving sleep.

The first time I tried yoga, I spent half the class worrying about whether my downward dog looked more like a limp cat. But once I got into the rhythm, I found it was the perfect way to unwind and connect with my body — especially when menopause had me feeling a little out of sync.

Cognitive Behavioral Therapy (CBT): A Mental Health Symptom-Relief Tool.

Cognitive Behavioral Therapy (CBT) is a beacon of hope for those experiencing menopause symptoms. It's talk therapy that focuses on changing negative thought patterns and behaviors. Widely used to treat conditions like anxiety and depression, it can also be a powerful tool for managing menopause symptoms, offering relief and a path to a better quality of life. However, it's important to note that CBT may not work for everyone, and, like any treatment, it has its limitations and potential side effects.

The Mechanisms Of CBT:

CBT equips you with practical strategies to manage anxiety, mood swings, and stress during menopause. You can learn to respond differently to menopause-related difficulties by identifying and addressing negative ideas. For instance, CBT can help you reinterpret your thinking and develop relaxation strategies to manage hot flashes more effectively, giving you a profound sense of empowerment and control.

CBT For Treating Sleep Problems:

One of the most valuable applications of CBT for menopause is treating sleeplessness. CBT for insomnia (CBT-I) is highly effective, emphasizing the modification of behaviors and ideas that support sleeping difficulties. Methodologies could call for cognitive reorganization, sensory control, and sleep limitation, which can provide hope and reassurance to those struggling with sleep problems during menopause.

I was astounded by the degree to which CBT improved my sleep problems. I used to lie awake for hours, wriggling and turning, my mind racing with concerns about everything from my job to whether I had remembered to water the plants. Following a few CBT sessions, I discovered how to calm my thoughts and design a genuinely effective evening ritual, which included journaling before bed and practicing progressive muscle relaxation, where I tensed and then relaxed each muscle group in my body. This process helped me release physical tension and unwind. I am sleeping now more peacefully than I have previously.

Limitations And Potential Side Effects Of Cognitive Behavioral Therapy (CBT) in Treating Menopause Symptoms:

Cognitive Behavioral Therapy (CBT) is increasingly recognized as an effective, non-hormonal treatment for managing menopause symptoms, particularly for mood swings, anxiety, and sleep disturbances. However, while it can be beneficial, there are limitations and potential side effects to be aware of:

Limitations of CBT in Treating Menopause Symptoms:

1. **Limited Effectiveness for Physical Symptoms:** CBT primarily targets emotional and psychological symptoms, so its ability to address physical menopause symptoms like hot flashes and night sweats is often limited. While it can help with the psychological response to these symptoms, it doesn't treat the root cause directly.

2. **Requires Active Participation:** CBT is a structured therapy that demands active patient involvement. For some menopausal women, finding the time, energy, or motivation to engage fully in regular sessions or homework assignments may be challenging.

3. **Delayed Results:** CBT is not a quick fix. It typically takes several sessions over a few months to see significant improvement in mood or sleep. Women seeking immediate relief may feel frustrated by the slower progress.

4. **Doesn't Address Underlying Hormonal Changes:** Since CBT focuses on the psychological aspects, it does not address the hormonal imbalances that cause many menopause symptoms. Women experiencing severe physical symptoms may need to

combine CBT with other treatments like hormone replacement therapy (HRT).

5. **Access to Qualified Therapists:** Finding a qualified CBT therapist with experience in menopause-related issues can be a challenge. Additionally, the cost of therapy may be prohibitive for some, and not all insurance plans cover mental health services like CBT.

Potential Side Effects of CBT:

1. **Emotional Discomfort:** Discussing deep-seated emotions, anxieties, or traumas during CBT can lead to temporary emotional discomfort. While this is part of the therapeutic process, it can be distressing for some women, particularly if they are already experiencing emotional volatility due to menopause.

2. **Over-reliance on Cognitive Techniques:** Some women may become overly reliant on CBT techniques and may neglect other forms of self-care, such as nutrition, exercise, or social support, which are also crucial during menopause.

3. **Frustration or Disappointment:** If expectations are not managed properly, some women may feel disappointed if CBT doesn't quickly or thoroughly alleviate all their symptoms. It can lead to frustration

and a sense of failure, especially if they hope for more immediate relief.

4. **<u>Relapse in Symptoms:</u>** Without continued practice of CBT techniques or refresher sessions, some women might experience a relapse in their anxiety, depression, or sleep disturbances once the therapy is completed.

5. **<u>Initial Increase in Sleep Problems:</u>** When CBT is used to address insomnia, sleep restriction techniques (such as limiting time in bed) can initially worsen sleep deprivation before leading to improvements. This phase can be frustrating and uncomfortable.

6. **<u>Possible Misalignment with Cultural or Personal Beliefs:</u>** CBT focuses on individual thought processes and may not align with everyone's cultural or personal beliefs about mental health and emotional well-being. Some may prefer alternative or holistic approaches over structured therapy.

7. **<u>CBT May Not Address Deeper Emotional Issues:</u>** While CBT is tremendous for symptom management, it doesn't always explore deeper emotional issues or past trauma, which may be contributing to the emotional challenges during menopause. For individuals needing a more in-depth exploration of emotional pain, additional types of therapy may be necessary.

All in all, while CBT can be a valuable tool for managing the emotional and psychological aspects of menopause, it's not a one-size-fits-all solution. It works best in combination with other treatments, lifestyle changes, and support networks to manage the full range of menopause symptoms. Understanding its limitations and potential side effects is crucial in setting realistic expectations and getting the most out of therapy.

Which Dietary Supplements Should One Try?

Dietary supplements promising to reduce menopausal symptoms abound on the market, but which ones are worth your time (and money)? The most often used choices are closely examined below:

1. **Calcium And Vitamin D:**

   These two nutrients, calcium and vitamin D, are crucial for maintaining bone strength, especially during menopause when the risk of osteoporosis increases. Calcium is an essential building block for strong bones, while vitamin D aids in its absorption. Whether from food, supplements, or a combination of both, aiming for 1,200 mg of calcium and 600–800 IU of vitamin D daily can help you take control of your bone health.

2. Magnesium:

Magnesium, a versatile mineral, plays a role in numerous bodily processes, including blood sugar management, muscle and nerve function, and bone health. It's also been linked to improved sleep and reduced anxiety, two common menopausal symptoms. By incorporating a supplement that provides 320 mg of magnesium into your daily diet, you can look forward to potential relief from these discomforts.

3. Omega-3 Dietary Acids:

Omega-3 fatty acids, found in fish oil and flaxseed, have been shown to reduce inflammation, promote heart health, and potentially lessen the severity of hot flashes. Aiming for a daily intake of 1,000 mg of omega-3s, you can take a proactive step towards managing your menopausal symptoms and improving your overall health.

4. Probiotics:

Gut health depends on these "good bacteria," which may affect everything from immune system response and digestion. Specific research indicates that probiotics could also aid weight control and lessen the severity of menopausal symptoms, including vaginal dryness and hot flashes. Search for premium probiotics with several strains and think about including foods strong in probiotics into your diet as well: yogurt, kefir, and sauerkraut.

Herbal Supplements:

- **Black Cohosh:** This widely used herbal remedy for menopause is believed to offer relief from mood swings, night sweats, and hot flashes. While it's important to be cautious, especially if you have a history of liver problems, the potential benefits of black cohosh can bring hope and optimism. Always consult your doctor and monitor any adverse effects.

- **Dong Quai:** Commonly known as "female ginseng," is used in traditional Chinese medicine to help balance hormones and alleviate menopausal symptoms. It's worth trying under physician supervision, even if some ladies find it beneficial while others discover nothing.

- **Ginseng:** Particularly helpful during menopause, ginseng is said to boost energy levels and fight tiredness. It is a flexible supplement for controlling a variety of symptoms as it may also aid with mood swings and sleep problems.

- **St. John's Wort:** Mostly regarded as a natural antidepressant, St. John's Wort could ease menopause-related mood swings and irritability. However, it's important to note that it can interact with certain drugs, such as birth control pills, antidepressants, and blood thinners. Before including it in your regimen, be sure to see your doctor to discuss any potential interactions.

Remember, you're not alone on this journey. Your healthcare provider is there to assist and advise you. So, if you're considering herbal supplements for menopause, be sure to consult with them first. This emphasis on professional support can help women feel cared for and less isolated in their menopausal experience.

Final Thoughts: Finding Your Way Through the Menopause Maze.

While the menopausal journey may seem complex, it's important to remember that you are in control. The key is to listen to your body and choose what's best for you, whether it's hormone replacement therapy, non-hormonal treatments, lifestyle adjustments, or a combination. Each woman's experience with menopause is unique, and there's no one-size-fits-all solution.

Try out various approaches and determine which one suits you best. If one approach doesn't yield the desired results, remember there are always other paths to explore. The key is to be kind to yourself, stay informed, and reach out for help when you need it. You don't have to face this alone. Remember that support is always within reach, whether it's heart-to-heart with your doctor, joining a support group, or simply talking to a friend over a cup of tea.

And remember, it's even better if you can find humor in the challenges. Menopause is an opportunity to embrace a new phase in life, armed with the knowledge and confidence to handle whatever comes your way, even if it brings unexpected changes. So, take a deep breath, wear comfortable clothes, and always remember — you've got this.

Checklist:

- ☐ Research non-hormonal medications or supplements for managing menopause symptoms.
- ☐ Try using vaginal moisturizers or lubricants if experiencing dryness.
- ☐ Explore mind-body practices like acupuncture or aromatherapy for relief.
- ☐ Please list supplements that might help and review them with your healthcare provider.

Action Plan:

1. **Non-Hormonal Medications:** Speak to your doctor about non-hormonal medication options for managing hot flashes or other symptoms.

2. **Vaginal Health:** If vaginal dryness is an issue, look into different moisturizers or lubricants and try them out.

3. **Mind-Body Techniques:** Commit to trying acupuncture, aromatherapy, or other alternative treatments for at least 2-3 sessions to see if they help.

4. **Supplements:** Review any dietary supplements with your doctor to ensure they are safe and effective.

10. What's True About Alternative Therapies?

"Menopause is proof that you can rise, no matter what life throws your way. You've survived, thrived, and now it's time to live fully." — Unknown

When you're going through menopause, it can be hard to find your way around the world of alternative treatments. Everybody has an idea, whether it's plant teas, yoga stretches, essential oils, or acupuncture needles. But what works, and what's just a clever marketing trick?

Here is a list of the most well-known herbs and what studies and real women say about them.

What Does and Doesn't Work for Herbal Remedies?

The Promise of Nature's Pharmacy: Herbal medicines are often the first choice for women who want to treat their menopause symptoms safely. It seems more relaxing to think about taking a pill made from flowers, roots, or leaves instead of a poisonous one. However, it's important to note that herbs, like any medication, can have side effects or interact with other medicines. Therefore, it's crucial to consult with a healthcare professional before starting any herbal remedy. There are also differences between herbs and how well they work for different people.

The Tried-and-True Ways.

1. Black Cohosh:

It is likely the most well-known plant used to help with menopause. People with hot flashes, night sweats, or mood swings are often told to try black cohosh. Some studies say it can work, especially in the short run, and other studies that say the benefits are minimal. If you try black cohosh, be sure to notice any side effects, especially if you already have stomach problems. Remember, your experience with black cohosh is unique to you, and it's okay if it doesn't work as expected.

When my hot flashes turned me into a walking torch, I tried black cohosh. Initially, I didn't notice a significant change, but my hot flashes seemed less severe after a few weeks. Was it the black cohosh, or was it just my body getting used to it? I didn't know, but I was ready to keep taking it.

Similarly, many women have found relief from their menopause symptoms with the help of herbal remedies. It's a journey of trial and error, but it's worth exploring if you're looking for a natural way to manage your symptoms.

2. Red Clover:

Red clover is another well-known crop that contains phytoestrogens, which are plant chemicals that mimic the effects of estrogen in the body. Some women swear by it to eliminate hot flashes and strengthen their bones. So far, though, the scientific evidence isn't all that clear. Some studies show little to no benefit. Red clover might be an excellent natural source of estrogen to try, but don't expect miracles.

3. Ginseng:

Ginseng is thought to help with tiredness, mood swings, and trouble sleeping. It can be beneficial during menopause because it helps your body deal with stress. The ginseng study looks good, especially regarding how it affects happiness and energy levels. However, as we've already said, results can differ for each person.

4. Valerian Root:

Valerian root is known to help calm people down, and it can help if menopause is making it hard for you to sleep. It won't make you sleep better, but it might help you get some much-needed rest.

5. Evening Primrose Oil:

This oil is said to help with breast pain and hot flashes because it is high in gamma-linolenic acid. While the effects may vary, most people find it safe to try, providing security and confidence in its use.

Herbs You Should Be Careful With:

- **Dong Quai:** Dong Quai keeps hormones in order in traditional Chinese medicine. It is also known as "female ginseng." However, most of the evidence for its success comes from anecdotes. Dong quai can be combined with some medicines, especially blood thinners.

- **Kava:** While some people believe that kava can alleviate nervousness and sleep problems, it's essential to be aware of its significant risk: potential liver damage. Before considering kava, it's crucial to discuss this risk with your doctor, as the damage to the liver can be severe.

- **St. John's Wort:** This herb, known for its potential to alleviate mild sadness, can also have adverse interactions with many medications, including birth control and antidepressants. It's not a standalone treatment for menopause, but if you're considering it for mood swings, professional advice is essential.

Herbal medicines are like friends who always set you up on blind dates because they want to help you. At times, it's a match made in heaven, and at other times, you wonder how you got sucked into it. If they're not "the one," don't hesitate to break up with them after a few dates.

The Controversy Over Bioidentical Hormones.

What Are Bioidentical Hormones? Bioidentical hormones are often sold as an "all-natural" option for hormone replacement treatment (HRT). They come from plant sources like soy or yams and are chemically similar to your body's hormones. It makes sense—why not replace what you've lost with something that fits perfectly?

The Good, the Bad, and The Myth.

- **<u>The Good:</u>** Some women say bioidentical hormones cause fewer side effects than manufactured ones. They can be custom-compound, meaning the dose can be tailored to fit your needs.

- **<u>The Bad:</u>** Custom-compound bioidentical hormones are not FDA-approved, so they are not controlled as strictly as regular HRT. This lack of regulation means there's potential for inconsistent dosages and impurities. Also, there isn't much long-term study on their safety and value, so the long-term risks are not well understood.

- **<u>The Myth:</u>** There isn't much scientific proof to support claims that bioidentical hormones are safer, more successful, or better than traditional HRT. Some experts say the benefits are primarily psychological and more the result of intelligent marketing than natural science.

When bioidentical hormones were first suggested to me, it felt like I was being offered a personalized solution. However, I learned that 'natural' doesn't always mean 'better.' I chose to stick with standard HRT, but I understand that every woman's journey is unique. Trust your instincts and do what feels right for you.

The Truth About Acupuncture And Other Holistic Approaches.

As a different way to treat menopausal symptoms, acupuncture and other holistic methods have become more popular. But do they work?

Is Acupuncture Based On Ancient Wisdom Or Modern Hype?

Acupuncture is an old practice in which thin needles are inserted into specific spots on the body to improve energy flow and keep the body's processes in balance. Some studies show acupuncture may help with mental issues, hot flashes, and even sleep problems. But the results aren't always great; how well they work depends on the practitioner's skill and how your body responds.

The Proof:

There is some hopeful but not conclusive research on acupuncture for menopause. Some studies show that it significantly reduces hot flashes and improves sleep quality, while others show that it doesn't work any better than a placebo. Further studies are required to grasp its effectiveness altogether.

The Experience:

Acupuncture is said to be very relaxing for many women, even though the science is still not sure about this. It's a nice break from the stress of menopause. You can lie down and let someone care for you for an hour.

I didn't believe in acupuncture at first, but after too many long nights, I chose to give it a try. I was surprised that after a few lessons, my night sweats improved, and I felt relaxed all around. Even though it wasn't a magic fix, I kept going back because it helped so much.

Other Holistic Methods.

- **<u>Aromatherapy:</u>**

  Lavender, peppermint, and clary sage essential oils are often used to ease the signs of menopause. With their unique properties, these oils offer a ray of hope in managing menopausal symptoms. Peppermint can help with hot flashes, lavender is relaxing, and clary sage is thought to keep hormones in balance. While there is little proof, the potential benefits of these oils can inspire optimism, especially if you enjoy their soothing scents. However, it's important to note that some people may be allergic to certain essential oils, so it's best to do a patch test before using them extensively.

- **<u>Massage therapy:</u>**

  Regular massages can be a powerful tool for stress relief, improved circulation, and muscle pain management, all common issues during menopause. More than just a treatment, it's a form of self-care every menopausal woman deserves. It's a way to pamper yourself and feel valued, acknowledging the importance of self-care in your menopausal journey.

- **<u>Healing with Reiki and energy.</u>**

The idea behind Reiki and other types of energy healing is that a practitioner can change the body's energy field to help with health and mending by using their hands. Some women say they feel more balanced and calmer after sessions, but it's important to note that little scientific evidence supports these claims. These treatments might help you feel better if you're willing to explore your spiritual side.

Phytoestrogens: Plant-Based Estrogens And Their Effects.

What Are Phytoestrogens?

Phytoestrogens, naturally occurring chemicals in plants, mimic the effects of estrogen in the body. They are present in various foods, such as flaxseeds, soy products, and beans. Many women opt for phytoestrogens over HRT, seeking a natural way to regulate their hormones.

What Are The Sources Of Phytoestrogens?

- **Isoflavones and Soy:** isoflavones are a type of phytoestrogen found in large amounts in soybeans. There are mixed results from studies examining how soy can help with hot flashes and bone health.

Women who live in countries that eat a lot of soy tend to have fewer menopause symptoms, but this could also be because of other things in their lives.

- **Flaxseeds:** Lignans, a different kind of phytoestrogen, are found in flaxseeds. Even though they're usually linked to gut health, there is some proof that they may also help with mild menopause symptoms.

Other Sources:

Plant-based foods like legumes, whole grains, and some veggies also have phytoestrogens, though not as much. Including these in your diet may be an easy and natural way to help your problems.

How They Work:

Phytoestrogens, by binding to estrogen receptors in the body, may offer a promising avenue for maintaining hormone balance. Some studies suggest that a diet rich in phytoestrogens could potentially reduce the frequency and severity of hot flashes, instilling a sense of hope for those experiencing menopause symptoms.

The Claim:

It's important to note that the effectiveness of phytoestrogens can vary from person to person. While some women report positive results, others may not notice significant changes. This variability is normal and should be considered when exploring natural hormone management options.

From my journey, I found that increasing my intake of phytoestrogens, mainly through tofu and flaxseeds, may have provided some relief. However, I also discovered that a diet rich in soy-based foods can become monotonous. This personal experience underscores the importance of finding a balance that works for you.

The Role of Essential Oils: Can Scents Make A Difference?

Aromatherapy, a form of alternative medicine, uses essential oils and concentrated plant extracts for medicinal reasons. The idea is that breathing in certain smells can change your mood, ease your symptoms, and make you feel better. In the context of menopause, aromatherapy can be a soothing and empowering self-care method. Lavender, peppermint, and clary sage oils are often suggested for menopausal women to help manage symptoms such as hot flashes, mood swings, and sleep disturbances and improve overall well-being.

How It Does (Or Doesn't) Work.

- **<u>Lavender:</u>** Lavender is helpful for sleep and rest because it is known to calm people down. It has mild effects on most women, but some find it helps with nervousness and mood swings.

- **<u>Peppermint:</u>** Peppermint oil is often used to treat hot flashes because it cools you down. Putting a few drops on the back of your neck or your arms can help for a short time.

- **<u>Clary Sage:</u>** This oil is often suggested for women with hot flashes or night sweats because it is thought to help balance hormones. There isn't much proof, but many women swear by it.

- **<u>Rose:</u>** The oil from roses is thought to improve mood and can be used to treat nervousness and sadness.

While essential oils may not completely alter your menopausal experience, they can enhance your well-being. Their pleasant scents can uplift your spirits, and their potential to alleviate symptoms is promising and provides a ray of hope in your self-care journey. Remember, they are not a substitute for medical care but a beneficial addition to your self-care routine.

Trying acupuncture for the first time is a bit like going on a blind date: you don't know what to expect, and things could go weird. It might be awkward, but it's worth it if it makes you feel better. Ensure that your practitioner knows the difference between a porcupine impression and a pressure point.

Aromatherapy Techniques: How to Use Essential Oils.

The good news is that essential oils are easy to use daily, even if you've never tried them. Before you start, here are some techniques to follow:

- **Diffusion:** Most people use essential oils this way. Putting a few drops of oil into a diffuser can fill the room with the smell of your choice. This is especially helpful for creating a calming environment before bedtime or setting a relaxing mood in your home office.

- **Applying To The Skin:** You can apply some essential oils directly to your skin, but mix them with a carrier oil first, like coconut or jojoba oil. To ease the signs of menopause, massage diluted lavender oil into your temples to get rid of headaches or put clary sage oil on your pulse points to control hot flashes.

- **Bath Soaks:** Putting a few drops of essential oils into a warm bath can make it feel like you're in a spa. Lavender and rose oils can help you relax, and peppermint and eucalyptus oils can wake you up.

- **Inhalation:** Consider the potential benefits of essential oils for a quick mood boost or to clear your mind. Whether you take them straight from the bottle or drop them on a cotton ball or paper, these oils, especially peppermint oil, could be a promising aid when you're tired or need help focusing.

How Well Do Essential Oils Work?

While the effectiveness of essential oils during menopause is not fully understood, many women report feeling calmer, more energized, or more balanced when using them. Aromatherapy can be comforting self-care practice, even if the effects are more about ritual and relaxation than the actual chemical properties of the oils.

At first, I needed clarification about essential oils. In other words, could a few drops of lavender help me sleep? But after a few nights of doing it, I did notice a slight change. I wasn't falling asleep like a baby, but I felt calmer and less antsy. I looked forward to the routine of setting up the diffuser and reading a book before bed almost as much as I looked forward to sleeping.

Caution In Using Essential Oils:

Despite their overall safety, it's crucial to be aware of the potential risks associated with essential oils. Skin irritations or allergic reactions can occur, especially if the oils are undiluted. Some oils, such as peppermint or eucalyptus, can be too potent for some individuals, leading to headaches or illness.

Additionally, certain essential oils can interact with medications or exacerbate certain health conditions. It's important to use them with caution and under the guidance of a healthcare professional to avoid these potential risks, ensuring your safety and peace of mind.

Finally, integrating essential oils into your menopause self-care routine can be a delightful way to nurture yourself during this transition. Taking a moment for self-care, such as deep breathing, relaxation, and reflecting on your well-being, can uplift your mood, even if it doesn't drastically alter your symptoms.

Remember, your well-being is a priority and finding scents that help you feel calmer and less anxious is empowering and a testament to your commitment to your health and control over your well-being.

Wrapping Up On Alternative Medicine.

When standard treatments don't work or don't appeal to you, alternative methods may help ease the symptoms of menopause. But going into these treatments with an open mind and a good dose of doubt is necessary. Herbal medicines, bioidentical hormones, acupuncture, and essential oils may work well for some women but not so well for others. Before starting a new treatment, remember that your unique journey and needs should guide your choices, and talking to a doctor is essential.

Each woman's experience of menopause is distinct, and solutions that are effective for one individual might not be suitable for another. This diversity is a beautiful aspect of this phase in your life, allowing you to explore, experiment, and find what makes you feel your best. Whether it's standard treatment, alternative therapies, or a combination of both, the most important thing is that you take care of your body, mind, and spirit.

Checklist:

- ☐ Research the effectiveness of popular herbal remedies.
- ☐ Talk to a healthcare provider about bioidentical hormones if you're considering them.
- ☐ Book an appointment with an acupuncturist to see if acupuncture helps with your symptoms.
- ☐ Identify any essential oils or holistic practices you'd like to try for symptom relief.

Action Plan:

1. **Research Alternative Therapies:** Read up on herbal remedies like black cohosh or evening primrose oil and decide if you want to try them.

2. **Bioidentical Hormones:** If considering bioidentical hormones, discuss with a trusted healthcare provider for their professional opinion.

3. **Holistic Treatments:** Try at least one holistic treatment (like acupuncture or aromatherapy) and note how it affects your symptoms.

4. **Essential Oils:** Experiment with essential oils (e.g., lavender for relaxation) to see if they improve your mood or sleep.

11. Menopause And Your Sexual Health.

"Don't let menopause hold you back. Keep reaching for your dreams."
— Unknown

During menopause, you may feel like things you used to take for granted are being stolen from you in the dark. The damage it does to your sexual health is one of its many heists that can feel very personal. It's okay to feel this way. But here's the thing: menopause doesn't have to end your sex life. It may change it, but it also presents an opportunity to rediscover and redefine intimacy in ways you hadn't thought of before.

Let's talk about what this stage means for your physical health and how to navigate it with ease, connection, and maybe even some humor.

Rediscovering Intimacy: How Menopause Affects Your Sex Life.

As estrogen levels drop during menopause, it's normal for your sexual desire to fluctuate. You may find yourself less interested in sex, and your vaginal tissues may become dry, making sex uncomfortable or even painful.

Remember, you're not alone in this experience. Many women go through these changes during menopause.

Understandably, many women report a decrease in sexual activity during menopause. However, it's important to note that regular sexual activity can help maintain vaginal health and reduce discomfort. The first step towards addressing these issues is understanding the underlying causes. This knowledge can empower you to take control of your sexual health and make informed decisions.

Here Are Some Of The Underlying Causes:

- **<u>Vaginal Dryness:</u>** Vagina dryness may be the most common complaint during menopause. When estrogen levels drop, vaginal walls become thinner and less flexible. This condition makes it dry and uncomfortable to have sex. It's like your body chose to make the Sahara Desert your new downstairs scene.

- **<u>Less libido:</u>** Changes in hormones can make you less interested in having sex. It's okay if you don't feel as 'in the mood' as you used to. This is a common experience during menopause, and you are not alone. Libido is a complicated thing that depends on hormones, feelings, and mental health. Stress, anxiety, and depression can all affect your libido, so it's important to consider your mental well-being when addressing changes in sexual desire during menopause.

- **<u>Physical Pain:</u>** Besides feeling dry, you may also feel pain in your body, like heat or itching, during and after sex.

Rewriting The Script:

First and foremost, it's important to remember that the changes you're experiencing are a normal part of menopause, and you're not alone in this journey. While it may feel like menopause has taken away your sexual drive, remember that intimacy is more than just sex.

This phase is a time to explore new ways to connect with your partner and strengthen your bond in ways that go beyond the physical. Embracing these changes can empower you, making you feel confident and in control of your sexual health.

- **Take Your Time:** Going through menopause means you should slow down in the bedroom. Don't rush through foreplay; take your time and try out different kinds of caress. Such engagement can help wake you up and ease your pain.

- **Lubrication:** It would help you buy a good-quality lube because it will immensely benefit you. It's okay to use it — consider it your new bedtime essential. What you do can make the difference between something painful and something enjoyable.

- **Use Vaginal Moisturizers:** These are different from lubricants because they're used all the time, not just during sex, to keep the vaginal tissues hydrated. Over time, they can help retain comfort and elasticity over time.

Sexual Confidence: Embracing Your Body And Desires.

One of the hardest things for women going through menopause is not being happy with their bodies. Your body can change how you feel about it, too. A drop in self-esteem can happen because of things like gaining weight, changing skin, and losing flexibility. But it's important to remember that your worth isn't based on your stomach, and your beauty isn't based on how stretchy your skin is.

- **Enjoy the Change:** Menopause is a time of change, and it's a chance to enjoy your body just as it is now. Enjoy the things that make you feel sexy, like a particular outfit, your underwear, or even just how your partner looks at you.

- **Redefine "Sexy":** It's not just about being young. It's about how you carry yourself and how sure you are of yourself. Menopause is a great time to change your ideas about what makes you sexy, using the things that make you feel strong and beautiful.

- **Explore Your Desires:** Now might be a good time to look into different parts of your sexuality. Without the stress of pregnancy, you can feel free in a new way. Being open to new experiences is essential, whether trying new things in the bedroom or focusing on your proximity to your mate.

When I reached menopause, there was a time when I looked in the mirror and didn't recognize the woman there. When I realized this was my new regular, I had to decide whether to be sad or happy about the changes. I bought new lingerie that I would not have been brave enough to wear in my 20s and chose to love my new curves. It's incredible how lace can make you feel better about yourself.

How To Make Your Relationship With Your Spouse Stronger.

Talking to each other is essential in any relationship, but it's even more important during menopause. Changes are happening in your body and feelings, and your wants may be different now than in the past. Letting your partner know about these changes is crucial so you can handle them together. This open communication can foster a deep sense of support and understanding, strengthening your bond during this phase of life.

- **Start the Talk:** Don't be shy about talking about how the menopause is making you feel physically and mentally. Maybe your partner doesn't fully understand what you're going through. It's up to you to tell them. It's not about whining but helping people understand and support each other.

- **Say What You Want:** Tell your partner what you want, whether it's more pre-play, lube, or more time. It would help if you also asked them what they need. Going through menopause affects both of you and being there for each other is an essential part of staying close.

- **Explore Together:** This phase in your life is an opportunity to experiment with new ways of being close to each other. To strengthen your relationship, use this time to try new things in the bedroom, cuddle up more, or engage in deeper conversations. Embracing these new experiences can bring a sense of excitement and hope to your sex life during menopause.

At first, I was afraid to tell my partner that I was going through menopause. But after a few awkward meetings where neither of us knew what the other needed, I realized the only way to move forward was to talk to each other.

We had a glass of wine, sat down, and talked it out. It was challenging, but it ultimately made us more resilient. We're back on the same team on this trip.

Remember that if you need help figuring out what's wrong, say it was the hormones. "Why did I cry during that ad?" Hormones. Why did I yell at you for no reason? Hormones. Why did I eat all the chocolate in the house? Hormones, for sure. But hey, at least we can blame something other than ourselves for a change, right? It's all part of the journey, so let's try to laugh about it together.

Pelvic Floor Health: Building A Stronger Base.

The pelvic floor is truly the hidden star of sexual health. These muscles help your bladder, bowels, and uterus stay in place and are vital for sexual health. These muscles can get weaker during menopause, which can cause problems like leakage and a loss of sexual desire. By taking care of your pelvic floor, you can regain control and enhance your sexual health, empowering you to enjoy a fulfilling sex life during menopause.

Why Pelvic Floor Health Is Important:

- **<u>Kegels Are Key:</u>** Kegel exercises can help you control your bladder better, make you feel more sexual pleasure, and even make your orgasms stronger. To do it, squeeze the muscles that you use to stop pee flow, hold for a few seconds, and let go. Do this several times every day.

- **<u>Pelvic Floor Physical Therapy:</u>** If you're having many problems, you might want to see a pelvic floor physical therapist. They can show you the proper routines and methods to strengthen these muscles and improve your general health.

- **<u>Benefits Beyond The Bedroom:</u>** A strong pelvic floor is good for your health in general, not just your sex life. It can improve your posture and core strength and even help prevent urinary incontinence. Regular pelvic floor exercises can enhance your overall flexibility and mobility, making everyday activities easier and more enjoyable.

While you wait for your coffee to brew, at the grocery store or during a Zoom call, you can do Kegels. They're like the secret workout you can do anywhere. Don't make that concentrating face, though, or people might start to wonder.

Wrapping Up: Taking Care of Your Sexual Health During Menopause.

Your sexual health may change during menopause, but it doesn't have to worsen. To get through this time with grace and confidence, you must be patient, creative, and kind to yourself. Menopause can be a chance to rediscover and change your sexuality. You can do this by being honest with your partner, trying out new ways of being intimate or taking better care of your body in new ways.

Don't forget that menopause is just a new part of your sexual life. Also, who knows? The freedom it gives might be the best one yet.

Checklist:

- ☐ Identify changes in your sexual health or desire.
- ☐ Try pelvic floor exercises to strengthen muscles and improve comfort.
- ☐ Have an open conversation with your partner about your needs and feelings.
- ☐ Research vaginal moisturizers or lubricants to enhance comfort during intimacy.

Action Plan:

1. **Pelvic Floor Health:** Start doing daily pelvic floor exercises to improve sexual comfort and function.

2. **Communicate with Your Partner:** By setting aside time for a candid conversation with your partner about how menopause is affecting your intimacy, you can foster a supportive and understanding environment.

3. **Try New Products:** Look into vaginal moisturizers and lubricants designed for menopause-related dryness. These effective products can help you feel more confident and comfortable during intimacy.

4. **Explore Intimacy:** Focus on non-sexual physical affection to maintain a connection while navigating changes in your libido. If you find it challenging to manage these changes, consider seeking professional advice from a healthcare provider or a sex therapist.

Part 3: The Emotional Side Of Menopause

12. How Menopause Makes You Feel.

"Menopause is a time for self-love and acceptance." – Anonymous

It's not just your body that changes during menopause; your emotions can also change a lot, making you feel like you're always on a roller coaster. You can go from laughing at something silly to crying over a dog food ad in the blink of an eye. To make it through this journey without losing your mind, you need to know why this happens and how to deal with it. Menopause can be hard on your emotions.

Let's talk about how to deal with the ups and downs with grace, self-compassion, and maybe even humor.

The Emotional Roller Coaster.

The mood changes that occur during menopause can be perplexing. When these feelings catch you off guard, it's easy to feel like you're losing control. But it's important to remember that you're not alone in this — it's all part of the normal process of menopause. These emotional shifts are a shared experience among many women, and understanding this can provide a sense of reassurance and solidarity, knowing that others are going through the same journey.

Why Do I Cry During Commercials?

- **Hormones on the Loose:** First, let's talk about those hormones. When your amounts of estrogen and progesterone change, they mess up the chemicals in your brain that control your mood. Serotonin, which is often called the "feel-good" hormone, can drop sharply during menopause, making you more likely to be sad, angry, and even cry over silly things.

- **Estrogen's Role:** Estrogen, an essential hormone in the female body, affects more than just your sexual health; it also changes how serotonin is made in your brain. When estrogen levels drop during menopause, serotonin levels fall, too. This decline can cause mood swings that seem to come out of nowhere. Understanding this hormonal shift can help you make sense of your emotional changes.

- **Crying As A Release:** It may be embarrassing to cry during an insurance ad, but tears are a standard way for your body to get rid of stress. Like a gas vent, you need to let it out occasionally.

One night, I was in tears watching an ad about a dog reuniting with its owner. I was sobbing into my teacup, wondering what was wrong with me. After a few similar incidents, I realized it wasn't the commercial; my emotions were having a rough day.

How To Cope.

So, what can you do when the tears won't stop? First, it's crucial to understand that this is a normal part of the process. Nothing is wrong with you; your body is adjusting to the new hormonal landscape. Be kind to yourself and allow your body the time it needs to adapt. Practicing self-compassion, a vital tool in navigating these emotional changes, can help you feel understood and less alone in your experiences.

- **Allow Yourself To Feel:** Don't hold your feelings inside. Permit yourself to cry if that's what you need. There are times when a good cry is just what you need to get your feelings out. Embracing your emotions and allowing yourself to express them is a form of self-compassion and acceptance, which is crucial during this phase.

- **Talk About It:** Sharing your experiences with someone you trust can be incredibly comforting. Whether it's a friend, a partner, or a doctor, opening up about your feelings can help you cope and make you feel less alone in your journey through menopause. It's important to remember that you're not alone in this, and sharing your experiences can help you feel more connected and less isolated, knowing that there are people who understand and support you.

- **<u>Practice Mindfulness:</u>** Mindfulness techniques, such as deep breathing or meditation, can help you stay grounded when your feelings get the best of you. These practices can help you focus on the present moment and reduce the impact of your emotions. Spending a little time daily on these techniques can make a big difference in managing your emotional changes during menopause. Additionally, engaging in regular physical activity, maintaining a healthy diet, and getting enough sleep can help regulate your mood during this time.

How To Deal With Anxiety: It's Not Just In Your Head.

The Anxiety Link:

Another common thing that goes along with menopause is anxiety. From mild fear to full-on panic attacks, it can happen at any time. Hormonal changes that cause other emotional signs can also cause panic attacks. Remember, these experiences are part of a normal process, and understanding this can help validate your feelings and reduce anxiety.

- **The Effects of Progesterone:** During menopause, your body makes less progesterone, which is supposed to calm you down. This decline can make you feel more tense and anxious.

- **The Fight-or-Flight reaction:** If you don't have enough progesterone to keep you calm, your body may respond more strongly to stress. It can trigger the 'fight-or-flight reaction,' a natural response to perceived threats. In simpler terms, even when there isn't a real threat, your body may react as if there is, leading to sudden worries and anxiety.

During my menopause, I experienced persistent worries that something was wrong, even when everything was fine. My heart would race in the middle of the night, and I was convinced I was having a heart attack. It took several visits to the doctor to realize that it was anxiety, a new and unwelcome presence in my life.

Strategies For Managing Anxiety:

Coping with anxiety during menopause requires a multi-faceted approach. Here are a few approaches that could be beneficial for you:

- **Stay Active:** Working out is a great way to deal with stress. It eliminates extra energy and produces more serotonin, which makes you feel better and lowers your stress.

- **Don't Drink Too Much Caffeine Or Alcohol**: Both can make your nervousness worse, so try to limit how much you drink, especially at night.

- **Learn How To Do Deep Breathing:** When you feel anxious, focus on your breath for a few moments. Inhale deeply through your nose, pause briefly, and then gradually exhale through your mouth. This action will help calm your body and mind and lower your stress.

- **Get Professional Help:** Don't hesitate to talk to a therapist or counselor if your worry is relentlessly affecting your life. Cognitive-behavioral therapy (CBT) and other types of treatment can significantly help people with worry.

Embracing The Mood Swings: Laughing (and Crying) Through It All

Riding The Emotional Waves:

Mood changes are one of the most well-known emotional effects of menopause. You may seem on top of the world for one minute and then snap at your family and friends for no reason the next. Rapid changes in hormone levels, especially estrogen and progesterone, are a big reason for these mood swings.

- **Estrogen's Role:** Estrogen plays a significant role in regulating mood. When estrogen levels fluctuate during menopause, it can lead to rapid changes in mood. It's not uncommon to feel a mix of emotions, from anger to sadness, all at once, sometimes within the same hour. Understanding this can help you treat yourself and those around you more kindly during these mood swings.

- **Self-Awareness:** Knowing that these mood swings are a normal part of menopause can help you treat yourself and those around you with a little more kindness during them.

I once laughed so hard at a joke that wasn't funny, then I started crying about ten minutes later because I had accidentally burned dinner. My husband wasn't sure if he should laugh with me or hide the sharp things.

How To Deal With Mood Swings:

Mood swings can be challenging, but there are ways to handle them:

- **Communication:** Tell everyone around you about what's going on. People close to you can help you deal with these mood swings by understanding.

- **Take A Break:** If you feel a mood swing coming on, let yourself leave the setting. Spending some time alone can help you calm down after a stressful event.

- **Keep A Mood Journal:** Write down your feelings every day. Tracking your moods can help you identify trends and triggers, which can be very helpful when dealing with and lessening mood swings.

Depression And Menopause: How They Affect Each Other.

Sadness is more than just mood swings. While mood swings are a normal part of menopause, it's important to recognize that sadness can be a symptom of a more severe condition. It's not just being sad; it's having a constant sense of fear, losing interest in things you used to enjoy, and being very tired all the time.

For some women, going through menopause can cause or exacerbate depression, which is a significant and often overlooked problem.

- **<u>Hormonal Imbalance:</u>** Menopause causes estrogen levels to drop, which can mess up the balance of hormones. This imbalance can affect brain chemicals like serotonin and dopamine, directly linked to mood control. In some cases, this can make you feel depressed.

- **<u>Changes In Your Life:</u>** Menopause often happens simultaneously with other significant changes, like when your kids move out, your parents get older, or you retire. These changes can also make you depressed.

Sometimes, during menopause, I felt like a shadow of the person I used to be. Things I used to enjoy, like gardening and reading, became less attractive, and I started to feel alone and cut off. It wasn't until I asked for help that I realized I had depression, which was a real problem that needed to be fixed.

Getting Help And Treatment.

If you suspect you might be experiencing depression, it's crucial to seek help. You're not alone on this journey. Here are some steps you can take:

- **<u>Talk To Your Doctor:</u>** Don't be afraid to talk to your doctor about your mental health. They can help you figure out if your symptoms are caused by menopause and offer treatments that will help.

- **<u>Consider Therapy:</u>** Cognitive-behavioral Therapy (CBT) and other types of treatment can help people who are depressed. Therapy can help you deal with your feelings and make your mental health better in general.

- **<u>Medication:</u>** Antidepressants may be needed to help keep your mood in check in some situations. It would help to talk to your healthcare provider about this before making this personal choice.

Self-Compassion: A Powerful Tool In Your Arsenal.

When you're going through menopause, your body is going through a lot of changes, and it's easy to start judging yourself. You may be angry at your body, impatient with your feelings, or think you're not handling things as well as you "should." This kind of situation calls for self-compassion.

- **What Does Self-Compassion Mean?** You should be kind, understanding, and patient with yourself, just like you would with a close friend. Realizing that you're having a hard time and that it's okay to fight is what it's all about.

- **Letting Go Of Perfection:** When you're going through menopause, it's helpful to let go of the idea that you must do everything correctly. Everyone has bad days, feels stressed, and doesn't always know what to do.

During a terrible day, I thought I should manage the situation more effectively. But then I stopped and asked myself, "Would I tell a friend who was going through the same thing?" Without a doubt, not. I would be kind to her, wait for her, and tell her she's doing a great job. At that point, I realized I needed to show myself the same kindness.

How To Develop Self-Compassion:

So, how can you develop self-compassion during menopause? The following are some of the few things you can do to make a big difference:

- **<u>Positive Self-Talk</u>:** Pay attention to how you talk to yourself, especially when things are hard. Change your negative, harsh thoughts to more positive and helpful ones. Saying things like, "I'm doing the best I can, and that's enough" instead of "I'm failing at this" can help. For instance, when you're feeling overwhelmed, remind yourself that it's okay not to always have everything under control.

- **<u>Mindful Acceptance</u>:** If you want to go through menopause, you need to be aware that the process takes time and that it's okay not to have everything under control. Mindfulness techniques can help you be in the present moment and accept what's happening without judging it.

- **<u>Treat Yourself Nicely</u>:** Allow yourself to enjoy things that make you feel good, like a long bath, a book, or a walk in the woods. These little ways to care for yourself can help you remember that you deserve care just like everyone else.

When you need to remember to be kind to yourself, picture giving yourself a pat on the back. Or, even better, picture your inner critic as a baby who is tired and cranky and needs a snack and a nap. Sometimes, just a little humor can change the way you see things.

Building A Support Network: You're Not Alone in This Journey:

Lastly, remember that being kind to yourself doesn't mean you have to go through menopause alone. Talk to your friends, join a support group, or find others doing the same thing. Sharing your journey with others can make it easier and give you a feeling of community.

Final Thoughts On Self-Compassion:

Going through menopause is very personal and unique. It's a time of change, growth, and sometimes challenges. Being compassionate toward yourself is the most crucial action you can take. Remember that you're not alone as you accept the changes and lean into the pain. Self-compassion isn't just a nice thought; it's an essential part of getting through this trip with strength and kindness.

Whenever I feel like I can't handle everything, I tell myself, "I am enough, just as I am." This simple but powerful phrase helps me stay centered and kind to myself all day.

With these tools and points of view, you can deal with the mental side of menopause with more kindness and understanding. Don't forget that it's okay to feel what you feel and to ask for help. After all, menopause isn't just a phase you have to get through; it's a part of your journey through life, and you deserve all the love and support you can muster.

Checklist:

- ☐ Track your mood changes to identify any patterns or triggers.
- ☐ Reach out to a mental health professional if you're struggling with anxiety or depression.
- ☐ Practice self-compassion during emotional lows.
- ☐ Consider trying Cognitive Behavioral Therapy (CBT) for mood-related symptoms.

Action Plan:

1. **Track Emotions:** Use a mood journal to note when you experience highs and lows, along with possible triggers.

2. **Seek Professional Help:** If emotions feel overwhelming, remember that you're not alone. Find a therapist experienced in menopause-related issues who can provide the support and guidance you need.

3. **Try CBT:** CBT is a proven method for managing negative thoughts and can be particularly effective for women experiencing menopause-related mood changes. Learn and experiment with CBT techniques for managing negative thoughts daily.

4. **Self-Compassion Exercises:** When feeling emotionally drained, remember that self-compassion techniques like positive affirmations or mindfulness meditation can provide comfort and relief. You have the tools to navigate these emotional lows.

13. Self-Care And Compassion.

"Menopause is a time for celebrating your achievements." – Anonymous

A woman's life changes a lot during menopause, and it's easy to forget about her own needs while she deals with the physical and mental changes. Self-care and kindness aren't just good ideas; they're necessary. Let's discuss what that means and how to make it happen, even when life gets too much.

Taking Time For Yourself: You Deserve It.

During menopause, one of the most important things I've learned is that taking time for myself isn't selfish; it's vital. It's easy to put yourself last when dealing with work, family, and everyday life. Right now, though, you need to place your health first.

Menopause can be very tiring. Your body is working too hard, and you constantly feel different emotions. Giving yourself time, even if it's just a few minutes with a cup of tea in the morning or the whole afternoon to do something you love, can help you recover and get back on track. It's about taking a break and breathe, bringing relief and comfort amid the storm.

To begin, set aside small amounts of time throughout the day. For example, you might meditate for 10 minutes in the morning or do something you've been putting off for an hour every Sunday afternoon. Consistence is vital; thus, taking care of yourself should be a regular part of your day.

I used to think self-care meant doing big, fancy things like going to the spa or a weekend trip. But I've learned that the little things are just as important during menopause. Now, I love going for daily walks in the area. They help me relax and enjoy the sunshine. It's a small thing that significantly affects how I feel. Other self-care activities could include reading a book, taking a warm bath, or practicing yoga.

Why Mental Health Is Important: Getting Help When You Need It.

Taking care of your mental health is an essential part of self-care, especially during menopause. Because of the changes in hormones, it's normal to have mood swings, worry, and even sadness. The important thing is to know when you need help, and it's okay to ask for it.

Menopause isn't just a physical change; it's also a mental one. A lot is happening in your brain, and you might feel stressed sometimes. Make sure you take care of your mental health and get help when you need it from a doctor, a support group, or even a trusted friend.

Make plans ahead of time, not when things go wrong. Talk to a mental health professional if you're feeling sad, nervous, or not like yourself all the time. Getting help is not a sign of weakness; it shows you are strong and in control. Remember that treatment isn't just for when things go wrong; it can also be used to keep your mental health in check before they do.

Initially, I was reluctant to attend therapy. I told myself, "I can handle this on my own," but the mood swings got too much for me, so I made an appointment. Talking to a professional helped me understand what I was going through and gave me ways to handle my feelings. Making that choice was one of the best things I have done for my mental health.

Humor As A Coping Mechanism: Finding The Funny Side Of Hot Flashes.

One thing that can help you get through the ups and downs of menopause is making jokes. It can help to find the funny side of things, like those sudden hot flashes that make you feel like you're standing in front of an open oven.

Laughter is a great way to release stress. It can quickly make you feel better and give you a break from all the stress in your life. Plus, it gives you a chance to meet other people who are going through the same thing. There's nothing better than bonding over a shared experience, especially one as uncertain as menopause. Humor can be a beacon of light in the darkness, lifting your spirits and giving you hope.

Begin by accepting the irrationality of it all. There will be weird and surprising times during menopause. Why not laugh at them? Another thing you can do is look for comedy that speaks to you, like a funny book, a stand-up show, or even just jokes about menopause (trust me, they're out there). Laughing with friends who understand what you're going through can also be very helpful.

I remember being in a meeting one time when, all of a sudden, I felt like I was in a sauna. My face turned bright red, and I could feel myself beginning to sweat. I didn't freak out; instead, I made a joke about how I was having my summer. It made an embarrassing situation funny for everyone. Laughter has become one of my favorite ways to get through hard times.

Here are some lighthearted menopause jokes to bring a smile to your face. Remember, laughter is the best medicine!

1. Ever found yourself bringing a fan to the grocery store? You're not alone! Menopause can hit anytime, anywhere, just like a 'flash sale'!

2. Menopause is like being a teenager all over again... Moody? Check. Hot all the time? Check. No idea what's happening with your body? Triple check!

3. I asked my doctor if my hot flashes would ever stop... He said, "Maybe in December, when it's freezing outside."

4. Why don't menopausal women play hide and seek? Because good luck hiding when you're radiating heat like a human furnace!

5. My husband asked why I was sitting in the fridge. I told him, "It's the only place where my internal thermostat makes sense!"

6. What's a menopausal woman's favorite exercise? An "internal" sprint! One minute she's fine; the next, she's running to open every window in the house.

7. Why did the menopausal woman start gardening? Because she finally understands what it's like to be surrounded by things that wilt unexpectedly! We're all in this together, ladies!

8. I told my husband I was going through "the change." He asked, "Into what? A dragon?"

9. How do you know you're deep into menopause? When you walk into a room, forget why, but get mad at everyone anyway!

What are your favorite menopause jokes? Please share them with other menopausal women, and let's keep the laughter going!

Stay Calm During Menopause.

It's essential to find ways to stay grounded during menopause when your body is undergoing many changes. Meditation and mindfulness are vital tools that help you stay calm, centered, and in charge, even when your emotions are trying to throw you off.

When practicing mindfulness, you don't have to worry about the future or feel bad about the past. It can help with physical problems like hot flashes and sleepiness and make you feel better and less stressed. Conversely, meditation stops your mind from talking all the time and helps you feel more at peace.

Meditation can be a simple and accessible tool for you; you don't have to do it for hours. Just sit quietly for five minutes daily and focus on your breath. If your mind starts to wander, slowly bring it back to the present moment. Over time, you can slowly make the period longer. Pay attention to everything you do, even just washing the dishes. It is what mindfulness is all about. Being fully present in the present moment is the goal.

At first, I wasn't sure if meditation would work for me. I didn't believe I could hold out for that much time. That said, it made me feel much more relaxed. It's now something I do every day, and it helps me start the day with a calm heart and a clear mind.

The Power of Nature: Why Being Outside Is Good for You.

Being outside makes everything better. Nature has a unique way of calming the mind, especially during menopause. It could be the fresh air, birds singing, or the feeling of the sun on your skin.

Going outside can help you feel better, lower stress, and improve your health. As a natural remedy for the stresses of modern life, it gives you a feeling of calm and perspective. Plus, it makes you want to be active, which is excellent for dealing with menopause symptoms. So, let nature be your guide, and let it inspire you to take that step outside, even when you don't feel like it.

Every day, go outside for at least a short walk. Enjoy parks, forests, and beaches if you can get to them. Don't forget to look up. Sometimes, looking at the clouds or the stars can help you see the bigger picture and feel more linked to the world around you.

I've always loved nature, but now that I'm going through menopause, I want to be outside more than ever. A walk in the woods helps me calm down and clear my mind. I always go outside when I feel stressed — my favorite way to relax.

Self-care and kindness are essential during menopause, and it's not enough to do something nice for yourself occasionally. It's about making changes that are good for your health, meeting your needs, and helping you handle this change with grace and strength. Don't forget that you deserve to take care of yourself.

When you do, you not only help yourself, but you also show others how to do it. Remember, self-care is not selfish. It's necessary for your well-being and your ability to navigate this significant life transition.

Checklist:

- ☐ Set aside time each day or week for yourself, whether it's a walk, a hobby, or relaxation.
- ☐ Practice mindfulness or meditation regularly.
- ☐ If you feel overwhelmed, reach out for support from friends, family, or professionals.

☐ Identify at least one self-care activity you can commit to regularly.

Action Plan:

1. **Daily Self-Care:** Commit to 30 minutes each day for an activity that brings you joy or relaxation.

2. **Practice Mindfulness:** Incorporate a mindfulness or meditation routine into your daily schedule (start with 5-10 minutes).

3. **Create a Support Network:** Make a list of people you can talk to about your situation and reach out when needed.

4. **Focus on One Habit:** Pick one self-care habit, like journaling or taking a nature walk, and make it part of your regular routine.

14. Relationship During Menopause.

"Menopause is a natural part of life, just like birth and growth." – Anonymous

Menopause is not just your journey but a shared experience with those around you. While it may present challenges in your relationships, it offers a unique opportunity for growth, understanding, and forging new connections. Let's explore how menopause can transform relationships and how to navigate them with honesty, kindness, and even a sense of adventure.

Talk To Your Partner.

When your partner doesn't fully understand what you're going through, menopause can make you feel alone. Communication — honest, open, and often — is critical to getting through this time together.

Changes in mood, energy, and intimacy during menopause can be confusing for your partner. By sharing your experiences, you can give them a deeper understanding of your journey, fostering a sense of mutual support and reassurance. This mutual understanding and support can strengthen your bond and make you feel more connected and cared for.

When discussing menopause with your partner, it's important to approach the conversation with a sense of calm and openness. Choose a time when you're both relaxed, and share what menopause is, how it's affecting you physically and mentally, and how they can support you. Remember, you're navigating this together; open communication is not just vital. It's empowering and helps you feel more in control of your journey.

Remember, not everyone will react positively or understand immediately. Be patient and give them time to process.

I remember the first time I tried to tell my husband about menopause. "I feel like I'm losing my mind!" I just blurted out because my mood swings and hot flashes were driving me a bit crazy. He inquired, "Can I help with anything?" His expression was vacant as he looked at me. That straightforward question opened the door to a more meaningful discussion. We now discuss it more openly, which has strengthened our bond.

Getting Support During Menopause.

During menopause, your friends can be helpful. They will listen to you without judging, and advice, or make you laugh when you need it the most. Your friends can be a great source of support, even if they aren't going through menopause themselves.

Having a strong group of people who care about you can help you get through menopause. It can make you feel less alone and more powerful to have friends who understand or are willing to learn what you're going through.

Feel free to ask your friends for help. Tell them about your problems, ask for help, and let them know how they can assist you. For instance, you could ask a friend to accompany you to a doctor's appointment or to help you research and understand the different treatment options. It can sometimes be very comforting to know that someone else gets it. Remember that friendship works both ways; help your friends through their struggles, whether they're going through menopause or something else.

Getting together with a group of pals for coffee once a month was one of the best things I did during menopause. It became a safe place to vent, share advice, and laugh at how silly it was. We called it our *'Menopausi-Queens*.' It was more than just a gathering; it was a shared experience, a sense of belonging, and a source of comfort. Knowing it was behind me made things a little easier.

Family Dynamics: Explaining Menopause To Kids And Loved Ones.

Women going through menopause aren't the only ones who can be affected by it. If you're having significant mood swings or changes in behavior, it can affect your whole family. It can help your kids, parents, or other loved ones understand what you're going through if you talk about menopause with them.

Some friends or family members may not react positively or understand immediately. Be patient and give them time to process. Your family may notice you're crankier, tired, or more sensitive than usual. They might take it personally or think something is wrong if you don't tell them why. By talking about menopause in a way appropriate for their age, you can help them see that it is a normal part of life and not something to be afraid of or dislike.

Talk about relevant things to their age and your connection with them. For younger kids, you could say that growing up means your body changes, which can make you feel different sometimes. You can go into more depth for teens and adults about the signs and what they can expect.

For instance, you could say, 'I'm going through a natural phase in my life called menopause. It's a time when my body is changing, and I might feel different than usual. But it's nothing to be scared of, and it's not your fault. I'm still the same person, just going through some changes. Trust your gut and let them know you're still the same person. You're just going through a phase.

I knew it was time to talk to my teen son when he asked me why I was "always in a bad mood." I told him that my body was going through menopause, which made me feel more tired or stressed out sometimes. He looked at me momentarily and then asked, "So it's like how my hormones make me cranky but yours are different?" I said, "Yes," and we both laughed. Even though it wasn't perfect, it helped him understand that it wasn't about him and it was just a part of what I was going through.

Dating And Menopause: Finding Romance During Midlife Changes.

Dating can be tricky when you're going through menopause. Whether you're in a long-term relationship or just starting to date again, the physical and mental changes that come with menopause can make you less confident and less interested in relationships. But it's also a time to be proud of who you are and create more profound and meaningful relationships.

Sometimes, menopause can make you feel less beautiful or desirable, which can affect your love life. The physical changes, such as hot flashes, weight gain, and vaginal dryness, can be challenging. But this time in your life also empowers you to redefine what love and closeness mean to you. The key is to find someone who appreciates you just as you are, with all your strengths and vulnerability.

If you're in a long-term relationship, it's crucial to be open with your partner about how menopause affects you and your body. Sharing your truth and your desires can make you feel heard and supported. Embrace this stage of life with all its challenges and uniqueness, knowing that love transcends physical desire. It's about connection, trust, and mutual respect; open communication is the key to maintaining these aspects of your relationship.

As I began dating again after getting divorced, I was worried about how menopause might change my love life. It was all I could think about — from having hot flashes on dates to how my body was changing. But I learned that being open and honest about where I was in life made the experience more authentic.

The right person will not only accept that you are going through menopause, but they will also value the strength and knowledge it brings.

Building A Support System: Finding Your Menopause Network

One of the most powerful things you can do during menopause is to surround yourself with people who care about you. These could be family, friends, healthcare professionals, or online groups where you can share your experiences and seek help. Having a community that understands what you're going through can be incredibly comforting and reassuring, making you feel less isolated and more connected.

If you try to go through menopause by yourself, it can be very lonely. People in your support system are there for you when things go wrong. They can give you advice, talk about their experiences, or listen when you need to vent.

First, think about the people you can lean on in your life. Talk to family or friends who have been through menopause and ask them what they think. Find support groups in your area, such as menopause support groups at your local community centers or online sites like Menopause Matters, where you can talk to people going through the same thing. Also, don't be afraid to get help from a professional, like a therapist, a menopause expert, or a doctor who can give you proper care.

I felt exhausted and a little lost when I first started having menopause symptoms. But when I talked to my friends and joined online groups, I realized I wasn't alone. It made me feel more connected and encouraged to share stories, tips, and even my complaints with others going through the same thing. It turned an experience that could have been very lonely into a journey everyone was on together.

Getting along with others can be challenging during menopause, but you can keep those ties strong and grow stronger with open conversation, a sense of humor, and a robust support system. Don't forget that this is a time of change and growth for you and the people in your life. Being honest and caring with each other during this time can make your relationships better and more connected than ever. Remember to care for yourself physically and mentally, which is crucial for maintaining healthy relationships.

Checklist:

- ☐ Have an open conversation with your partner about how menopause affects your relationship.
- ☐ Lean on your friends for support and connection during this time.
- ☐ Explain menopause to your children or loved ones, if necessary, in a way that fosters understanding.
- ☐ Take time to nurture your existing relationships, even as you focus on your health.

☐ If dating, be honest with potential partners about your needs and experiences.

Action Plan:

1. **Open Dialogue with Your Partner:** Set aside a time for an honest conversation about how menopause has affected your emotional and physical intimacy.

2. **Lean on Friends:** Schedule regular catch-ups with friends to share your experiences and get the support you need.

3. **Explain Menopause to Family:** Create a simple way to explain your menopause symptoms to children or other family members so they better understand what you're going through.

4. **Dating:** If dating, be open with potential partners about the changes you're experiencing so you can set expectations and maintain open communication.

5. **Nurture Relationships:** Make a conscious effort to maintain and strengthen your connections with friends and family, even as you prioritize self-care.

15. Menopause And Career.

"Don't let menopause hold you back. Keep reaching for your dreams."
— Unknown

Menopause changes your personal life and can significantly impact your job. Many women navigating menopause at work face challenges that can affect their work, relationships with coworkers, and overall job satisfaction. However, with the right strategies, you can overcome these challenges and continue to excel in your work, showcasing your resilience and adaptability and feeling empowered to manage these changes.

Workplace Challenges: Navigating Menopause At Work.

During menopause, the job can be challenging. You must deal with hot flashes, brain fog, and mood swings while also making goals and taking care of your responsibilities. When you add the stress of keeping up a business appearance, it's easy to see why many women find this period especially hard. These symptoms can affect your job performance, making it crucial to find effective coping strategies.

Physical Challenges:

Dealing with hot flashes is one of the most common problems people face at work. Let's say you're giving a talk when you suddenly feel like you're in the Sahara Desert. You're desperately trying to keep your cool physically and figuratively as the sweat starts to pour out. It can be not very pleasant and make you feel less confident.

I had a hot flash once during an important client meeting. As my face turned bright red, I could only think, "Please don't notice, please don't notice." Of course, everyone did notice. "Hey, that's definitely a unique approach to spice things up in a negotiation!" I ended up making a joke about it. It made people feel better, showing how random and bothersome these symptoms can be.

Cognitive Challenges:

Menopause can also affect brain function, causing what is commonly known as "brain fog." It can manifest as trouble focusing, forgetfulness, or difficulty finding the right words. It can make you feel like you're not doing your best at work when things are moving quickly.

Emotional Challenges:

The mood swings that come with menopause don't end when you leave the office. You can bring your mood swings, anger, and stress to work with you. You could yell at a coworker or feel incredibly stressed out about things that used to be easy for you.

How To Manage Things:

Recognizing these problems is the first step in dealing with them. Don't be hard on yourself if you need a break or have a day off.

Here are some ideas that could work. Acknowledging and addressing these issues makes you feel understood and supported in your workplace.

- **Layered Clothing:** If hot flashes bother you, wear clothes that aren't too tight or loose so you can change them as the day goes on. Keep a small fan at your desk or use a cooling towel to manage sudden heat waves.

- **Drink Plenty Of Water:** Drinking enough water can help keep your body temperature in check.

- **Use Technology:** Use digital tools like to-do lists and notes to clear your thoughts and stay on top of things.

- **<u>Take Breaks:</u>** If you need to clear your mind, don't be afraid to leave your work briefly. Remember, taking care of yourself is not a sign of weakness but a necessity during this challenging time.

How To Talk To Coworkers: Breaking The Silence.

The shame and silence that surround menopause are two of the hardest things to deal with at work. Many women don't want to talk about their symptoms with coworkers or bosses because they're afraid it will be seen as a sign of weakness or that they will be treated differently.

Addressing the silence surrounding menopause in the workplace is essential for the well-being of all individuals and for creating a more supportive environment for women. By encouraging open communication about menopause, we can make a workplace where everyone feels comfortable and less isolated.

Start by deciding how much and who you want to share with. You don't have to tell everyone, but it might help to tell your boss or the HR department, especially if you need accommodation, like changing the temperature in your office or having flexible work hours.

- **<u>Talking to Your Manager:</u>** When you talk to your manager about menopause, focus on how your symptoms affect your work and what changes could help you be more efficient. For instance, if you have trouble with hot flashes, you could ask for a fan or a less strict dress code.

- **<u>With Coworkers:</u>** You can keep things light with coworkers. Explaining something as easy as "I'm going through menopause, that's why I seem a little off" can help people understand.

Being honest with my coworkers made a big difference for me. I stopped trying to hide my symptoms and started saying things like, "Excuse me, I'm having one of those brain fog moments that come with menopause. Please bear with me!" I was able to connect with other women going through similar situations, and that helped ease my anxiety. We made a support group out of nothing, which was very helpful.

How To Balance Your Health And Career: Strategies For Success.

It would be best to keep your job and health in check during menopause. It's about finding the right mix between doing your job and caring for yourself. You may need to change some things about your work, but that doesn't mean you must give up your career success.

Put Self-Care First.

One of the most crucial steps you can take is to prioritize self-care. This includes ensuring you get enough sleep, eat healthily, exercise, and take time to relax. By prioritizing your physical and mental well-being, you can enhance your job performance and feel more valued in your workplace.

Flexible Working Arrangements.

Suppose your boss lets you ask for open work hours. You could request to work from home when things are callous, change your hours to suit your energy levels better, or even reduce your workload temporarily if necessary.

Managing Your Time.

Managing your time well can also help you balance work and health. Divide your work into manageable tasks, and don't be afraid to ask for help when needed. Use schedules, apps, and plans to keep track of your tasks and ensure everything gets noticed.

Seeking For Help.

When you're struggling, don't hesitate to seek help. Whether it's talking to a therapist specializing in menopause, joining a support group, or consulting a menopause specialist, reaching out for support can make you feel less isolated and more connected during this challenging time.

How To Make The Workplace More Supportive.

Lastly, try to make the workplace a good place to be. If you're a leader, you might want to make rules that help women going through menopause, like letting them set their hours and giving them access to health tools. You could also encourage open conversations about menopause at work.

It took some time to learn how to balance my health and work during menopause. I understood I had to pay attention to my body and make changes so I could not just push through my problems. By putting myself first and telling my boss what I was going through, I could keep up my work performance without risking my health. It was worth it, even when it wasn't easy.

Dealing with menopause at work isn't easy, but it's possible to keep doing well in your job if you have the right tools and a supportive environment. By facing problems head-on, being honest with coworkers, and finding a good balance between work and personal obligations, you can get through this part of life and use it to grow and succeed in your career. Remember, you are not alone facing this situation. Many other women are, too, and if we all work together, we can make the workplace a better place for everyone.

Checklist:

- ☐ Evaluate how menopause symptoms have impacted your work performance or energy levels.
- ☐ Implement workplace accommodations (like flexible hours or a fan) to improve comfort.
- ☐ If necessary, communicate with your manager or HR about accommodation or support you may need.
- ☐ Create a work-life balance plan that includes stress management techniques.
- ☐ Look for support networks within your industry or community for menopausal women.

Action Plan:

1. **Assess Impact on Work:** Consider how menopause symptoms may be affecting your productivity or mood at work and write down specific challenges.

2. **Workplace Adjustments:** Identify small changes that can make your work environment more comfortable, such as having a fan at your desk or taking breaks to relax.

3. **Open Communication:** Consider talking with your HR department or manager about any adjustments or accommodations that could

help. This open dialogue will ensure that your needs are heard and understood, fostering a supportive work environment.

4. **Work-life balance:** Create a plan that includes time for stress-relief activities, such as exercise, mindfulness, or hobbies. This will help you manage work demands alongside menopause, providing a sense of relief and control over your life.

5. **Seek Out Industry Support:** Research women's groups or menopause-specific support networks within your field or community to find solidarity and shared experiences.

Part 4: Life Beyond Menopause

12.   The Postmenopausal You.

"You are not a victim of menopause. You are a conqueror." – Unknown

Menopause is not the end but the beginning of a new chapter. With your hormones leveling off, you can focus on what truly matters. As you adapt to your new routine and prioritize your health, happiness, and future, the post-menopausal years can be some of the most fulfilling and rewarding. It's a time of freedom, self-discovery, and personal growth.

Getting Used To The New Normal: What To Expect Going Forward.

The first thing you should know about going through menopause is that your body has adjusted to its new hormone levels. The changes in estrogen, progesterone, and testosterone have stopped going up and down. It means that the worst of your hot flashes, night sweats, and mood swings are probably over.

But that doesn't mean everything will be easy — new changes and problems exist.

Physical Changes.

Your body may feel different in small or big ways. Your metabolism might slow down, making it easier to put on weight and more challenging to lose it. Your skin may feel dry, and your hair may start to thin. You may still feel dry in the uterus, and your bones may become less dense, which raises your risk of getting osteoporosis.

Changes In Your Emotions.

When it comes to emotions, postmenopause can be a mixed bag. On the one hand, many women say they feel a sense of freedom and relief because they no longer have to deal with periods, PMS, or hormonal swings. However, you may feel lost or unsure of what to do next. There's nothing wrong with missing the woman you used to be, but this is also a chance to change who you are.

After realizing the hormonal chaos was over, I remember feeling calm in a way I hadn't felt in years. But a thought also didn't go away: "Now what?" I hadn't given much consideration to what would follow menopause since I was primarily focused on just getting through it for so long. After a while, I started to see menopause as a fresh start — a chance to focus on myself for a while.

Health Considerations: Taking Care of Your Bones, Heart, and More.

Now that you're past menopause, taking care of your health is more important than ever. Estrogen loss can affect many body parts, so keeping up with your health is essential.

Bone Health:

Loss of estrogen can make you more likely to get osteoporosis because it helps keep bone mass up. Get enough calcium and vitamin D to keep your bones strong and do weight-bearing activities like dancing, walking, or strength training.

Heart Health:

Menopause can also hurt your heart. As estrogen levels drop, the chance of getting heart disease increases, so monitoring your blood pressure, cholesterol levels, and general heart health is essential. Eating heart-healthy diet, working out daily, and dealing with worry are all very important.

Regular Medical Checkups:

Regular medical checkups are crucial at this stage of life. Don't skip those mammograms, bone density tests, and cholesterol checks. They're more important than ever. By staying on top of your health, you can catch any potential problems early, providing you with the security and care you need.

After menopause, I paid a lot more attention to my health. I began taking calcium vitamins, worked out more regularly, and made sure I kept all of my medical appointments. Taking care of my health now would pay off in the long run, even though it wasn't always easy, especially when my life got busy.

Finding Joy And Purpose: It's Time To Focus On You.

One of the best things about postmenopause is that it gives you time to focus on yourself. You now have the time and energy to rediscover what makes you happy and gives your life meaning. If you've been a parent, the pressures of raising a child are likely to ease, and your job may be entering a more stable phase.

Reassessing Priorities:

Now is a great time to look back on your life. Which things, people, or goals are most important to you? Have you ever meant to do something but never found the time? Now that you're past menopause, you can put these things first.

Exploring New Interests:

Many women use this time to try out new hobbies or interests. Whether you want to learn a new language, play an instrument, travel, or participate in community events, the options are endless. Another thing that many women start to think about at this point is how they can give back, whether through teaching, volunteering, or just spending more time with family and friends.

Setting New Goals: Embracing Inspiration and Motivation.

Feel free to make new goals, big or small. You might have wanted to write a book, plant a yard, or run a race for a long time. Now is the time to get that thing you want. Setting and reaching new goals can give you a new sense of meaning and happiness.

That book I had been thinking about writing for years finally got written for me after menopause. I also learned to garden, now one of my biggest loves. Caring for plants and watching them thrive brings a great sense of fulfillment. It reminds me that I can keep growing and doing well no matter how old.

Redefining Beauty And Aging: Getting Older With Grace.

You don't have to try to look like you're still in your 30s to age naturally. You can find beauty in every stage of life and accept the changes that come with getting older. A lot of the time, people think that beauty and youth go hand in hand, but that's not true. Natural beauty comes from being sure of yourself, accepting yourself, and having the knowledge that only comes with age.

Appreciating Your Body:

Your body has seen and done much as it has brought you through decades of life. You should love and appreciate it. Don't think about the lines, grey hair, or extra weight on your body. Instead, think about what it can still do. Be proud of your body's stories and how strong and resilient you are.

Redefining Old Age:

Redefining getting older is a powerful act of self-empowerment. It's about not letting your age define or stop you from reaching your goals. You're not 'over the hill,' you're atop the hill, where the view is better and bigger than ever.

Care for Yourself and Beauty Routines:

Caring for your body, hair, and face can make you feel great regardless of age. But taking care of yourself isn't just about how you look; it's also about feeding your soul. You can age gently by taking care of yourself. This could mean taking a relaxing bath, going to the spa, doing what makes you happy, or even practicing mindfulness or meditation. The secret is to identify and include enjoyable things in your daily routine.

I used to worry a lot about getting older, but going through menopause has helped me change how I feel about it. I love the laugh lines around my eyes because they mean I've lived a happy life. I love my silver hair, which makes me feel wise. To me, aging means living a whole life and welcoming every stage with open arms.

Reinventing Yourself: Discovering New Passions And Hobbies.

The years after menopause are a time to embrace new experiences. With fewer tasks and more time for yourself, it's a great time to discover new hobbies and interests that will add joy and satisfaction to your life.

Try New Things:

Feel free to try something new and leave your comfort zone. Many things can come from trying new hobbies, like drawing, learning to play the piano, or even writing a blog. You should be curious and open-minded when you try new things because you never know what might spark a new interest.

Finding A Community Of Like-Minded People:

Many hobbies and interests have communities of people who share them. Finding a community, like a book club, a gardening group, or a fitness class, can help you make friends and feel like you belong. It's a beautiful opportunity to connect with others who share your interests and understand your journey.

Pursuing Lifelong Learning:

Learning continues as you get older. After menopause can be a great time to return to school, start a new course, or keep learning. Whether you attend school, take online classes, or study independently, learning new things and growing can keep your mind and spirit sharp.

On the spur of the moment, I chose to take a photography class after menopause. I loved taking pictures as a child but never knew how to do it right. I enrolled in a class that exposed me to an entirely different world. I became interested in recording the beauty of everyday life through my lens. It's more than just a hobby for me now; it helps me see things differently.

The years after menopause are a time of change. Embracing this stage of life can be very beneficial as you get used to the new normal, take care of your health, and find joy and meaning in your life. It is what postmenopause is all about: changing how you look, how you act, and what it means to live a whole and happy life. There is a new beginning, not just a finish. The best part is that you get to write the story. Remember, maintaining a healthy lifestyle, including regular exercise, a balanced diet, and regular health check-ups, is crucial in this stage of life.

Checklist:

- ☐ Create a list of new hobbies or activities you'd like to explore post-menopause.
- ☐ Reflect on the lessons you've learned throughout your menopause journey.
- ☐ Set new health and wellness goals to maintain your physical and emotional well-being.
- ☐ Consider taking a class or pursuing a new passion that excites you.
- ☐ Stay connected to a community or support group that understands your experiences.

Action Plan:

1. **Explore New Hobbies:** List activities or passions you've always wanted to explore and commit to trying one this month.

2. **Reflect on Your Journey:** Take some time to journal about how menopause has shaped you and the lessons you've learned along the way.

3. **Set New Wellness Goals:** Create a health plan that includes regular exercise, a balanced diet, and mental wellness practices to help you thrive in this new chapter of life.

4. **Pursue Passion Projects:** Sign up for a new class, hobby, or activity that excites you and gives you a sense of purpose and joy.

5. **Stay Connected:** Connect with women who share similar experiences through online communities or in-person groups to continue feeling supported and understood.

17. Dispelling Menopause Myths.

"Menopause is a badge of honor, a testament to a woman's journey."
- Anonymous

Even though menopause is a normal part of a woman's life, many myths and false beliefs about it can make it seem strange or even scary. Most of the time, these myths come from cultural stereotypes, out-of-date medical knowledge, and media portrayals of women that don't match up with how they live. By dispelling these myths and replacing them with facts, we empower ourselves with knowledge and understanding, instilling confidence and control.

Debunking Common Misconceptions: What You've Heard vs. What's True.

Dispelling common myths about menopause is crucial, as it empowers women with accurate information and dispels fear. Let's replace what you've heard with what's real.

Myth #1: Menopause Only Happens To Women In Their 50s.

Many people think that women in their 50s are the only ones who go through menopause. The average age of menopause is about 51, but it can happen to different women at different times. Some women go through menopause in their early 40s or even late 30s. It is called early or premature menopause. Other women don't go through it until their late 50s or even early 60s. There is no set time for menopause that works for everyone, and each person's experience is unique and valid.

It shocked me when a friend of mine started showing signs of menopause when she was in her late 30s. It woke me up to the fact that menopause doesn't happen on a set schedule — each person goes through it differently. I remember feeling scared and confused when I first started experiencing menopause symptoms but learning about my friend's experience helped me realize that it's a normal part of life and that I wasn't alone. I also remember feeling relieved when I learned that menopause doesn't mean the end of my sexual life and that there are ways to manage the symptoms.

Myth #2: Menopause Marks the Conclusion of Sexual Life For Women.

A common false belief about menopause is that it means the end of your sexual life. It's just not true. Menopause can make your sex life different, like making your vaginal area dry or lowering your libido, but that doesn't mean you can't have sex anymore.

After menopause, many women find that their sex lives get better because they don't have to worry about birth control and may feel better about their bodies. So, there's no need to worry; your sexual life can continue and even improve after menopause.

Myth #3: Menopause Makes You Gain A Lot Of Weight.

By dispelling this and other myths about menopause, you can take control of your health and well-being, feeling empowered and informed about the changes your body is going through.

It's normal to hear that women who are going through menopause will gain a lot of weight. Changing hormones can cause changes in body makeup, like putting on weight around the middle, but that doesn't mean you'll gain a lot of weight. Diet, exercise, and how you deal with stress are all significant parts of how your body changes during menopause. At this point in life, staying busy and eating well can help you keep the weight off.

Myth #4: Hot Flashes Are the Only Symptom of Menopause.

Hot flashes are often the first sign that someone is going through menopause. However, they're not the only sign. Each woman's experience is unique, with some having many signs and others having few. Understanding the individuality of these experiences can make you feel more understood and less alone in your journey, providing a sense of reassurance and relief.

Myth #5: Hormone Replacement Therapy (HRT) Is Dangerous.

While it's true that hormone replacement therapy (HRT) has some risks, it can also be a beneficial option for managing severe menopause symptoms. The key is to seek professional advice from your healthcare provider, who can guide you through the risks and rewards specific to your case. It's important to remember that HRT is not the only option, and there are other ways to manage menopause symptoms. Your healthcare provider can help you decide what's best for you.

I was scared to even think about HRT for a long time because of all the bad things I had heard about it. But after doing some study and talking to my doctor, I saw that the pros might be more excellent than the cons for me. Things are different for everyone, and you should choose based on facts, not fear.

The Cultural Perspective: How Different Cultures View Menopause.

Menopause affects women all over the world, but how it is seen and dealt with changes a lot from one culture to the next. Menopause is seen as a normal and even a welcomed part of life in some cultures, but in others, it may be looked down upon or feared. For example, in some African cultures, menopause is a time of celebration and transition. In contrast, in some Western cultures, it is often viewed as a medical condition that needs to be controlled or treated. In Japan, menopause is usually seen as a regular part of aging that makes you wise and respectful, and Japanese women often report fewer menopause symptoms.

Western Perspectives:

Menopause has long been seen as a medical condition that needs to be controlled or treated in many Western countries. People tend to focus on the wrong things about getting older — like hot flashes, mood swings, and getting older — rather than the good things. This way of thinking can make women going through menopause feel anxious or not good enough.

Eastern Perspectives:

Many Eastern cultures, like Japan and China, see menopause as a regular part of aging that makes you wise and respectful. Japanese women, for example, often say they have fewer menopause symptoms. It could be because of cultural beliefs that don't view this time of life negatively. "Konenki," the Japanese word for menopause, means "renewal years" or "years of energy," which suggests a more positive attitude.

Indigenous Perspectives:

In some Indigenous countries, older women, even those who have gone through menopause, are seen as wise and strong leaders. As they enter menopause, women take on new moral and social duties, which is seen as the start of their new role as matriarchs or elders.

Learning about how people in other countries view menopause changed how I felt about my own. It made me understand that the society we live in shapes how we see things and that there is no "right" way to think about menopause. Our personal experiences and feelings genuinely matter and should guide how we navigate menopause.

Menopause In The Media.

How we think about menopause is primarily shaped by the media, which hasn't always been helpful. Women going through menopause were either ignored or made fun of in pop culture for a long time. For example, shows often use hot flashes and mood changes as comedy fodder. But the story is slowly beginning to change.

In the past, the media has often shown menopause in a bad light. Women who are going through menopause are frequently portrayed as "hormonal," illogical, or too sensitive. Women may feel wrong about what they're going through because of these harmful beliefs. Plus, the fact that older women aren't shown much recognition attest to the idea that they aren't seen or deemed important anymore.

However, in the past few years, the media has been showing menopause in a more upbeat and accurate way. This shift in media representation is a hopeful sign, as it brings older women's problems, like menopause, to the public's attention in a more respectful and understanding manner.

For instance, talk shows and documentaries are starting to talk about menopause more openly, featuring real women from diverse backgrounds sharing their experiences and experts providing valuable insights. This positive change in media portrayal is evident in shows like 'The Golden Girls' and 'Grace and Frankie, 'and movies like 'Hot Flash' and 'Menopause: The Musical, 'which depict menopause in a way that instils hope and optimism.

For example, 'The Golden Girls' often addressed menopause as a natural part of life, and 'Grace and Frankie' portrayed menopause as a topic of open discussion among friends rather than a taboo. These portrayals help make the topic more normal and less stigmatized.

Menopause isn't always a laughing matter, but finding humor can help you cope. Many entertainers are now talking about menopause in funny and realistic ways, not to belittle women's experiences but to provide a light-hearted perspective that can help take some power away from our fears and worries.

We can laugh at the silly things that happen, like trying to fan yourself with a magazine during a hot flash, and in doing so, we can find strength and resilience in the face of change. This positive approach to menopause can help women feel more empowered and less stigmatized.

I used to cringe at the way menopause was portrayed on TV, but now I find myself seeking out shows and movies that tackle it with humor and honesty. It's refreshing to see my own experiences reflected on me in a way that feels real rather than exaggerated for laughs. This validation and understanding through humor and honesty is a powerful tool in changing societal attitudes towards menopause.

Historical Views on Menopause: How Our Understanding Has Evolved.

Over the ages, we've learned a lot about menopause, but it hasn't been easy. Menopause has been misread and mistreated in the past, with women's experiences being ignored or seen as signs of a problem.

Ancient Views:

In the past, some people thought that menopause was a sign that a woman was getting older, reflecting how society generally felt about aging. Some countries thought that women who had gone through menopause were sage, while others looked down on them or even feared them. Before now, doctors didn't know much about menopause, so women often used local medicines or spiritual practices to deal with their symptoms. These practices included black cohosh, Dong Quai, rites of passage, shamanic healing, soy-rich diets, massage and bodywork., believed to alleviate symptoms like hot flashes, insomnia, and mood swings.

Menopause In Ancient Time:

In the 1800s and early 1900s, menopause was often seen as a medical condition. Sometimes, women were given iffy treatments, like hormone shots made from animal products, or they were even given surgeries, like hysterectomies. A common belief was that menopause made women insecure and unfit for their social jobs. This belief reinforced harmful stereotypes.

What We Know Now:

It wasn't until the second half of the 20th century that doctors learned more about menopause. In the 1960s, Hormone Replacement Therapy (HRT) was created, which was a big deal because it gave women a way to deal with their problems. HRT involves replacing the hormones that the body stops producing during menopause, which can help alleviate symptoms like hot flashes and mood swings.

However, it led to discussions about the pros and cons of medical interference with a normal process. Today, menopause is seen as a normal part of life, and more and more attention are being paid to personalized care, informed choice, and all-around methods of handling symptoms. HRT, along with other treatments like lifestyle changes and alternative therapies, is one of the options available for managing menopausal symptoms. This focus on individual needs and preferences and the empowerment it brings makes women feel valued and respected in their menopausal journey, fostering a sense of worth and respect.

Knowing about the history of menopause helped me see how far we've come. There is still work to be done to educate and raise awareness, but I'm glad we live in a time with more choices and tools to help us get through this part of our lives.

The progress in menopause research and treatment has given us more options and control over our menopausal journey, instilling a sense of confidence and empowerment. We now have a better understanding of menopause and more effective treatments, giving us the power to navigate this phase of our lives with confidence and control.

Misconceptions and myths about menopause can make this time in your life seem scary, but knowing the facts gives you power. By debunking these myths, we can empower ourselves and take control of our menopausal journey, instilling confidence and control. It's not just a time of change; it's a time of strength, and every woman should know the truth before she goes into it. This knowledge can empower you, giving you the confidence and control you need to navigate this phase of your life.

Checklist:

- ☐ Identify common menopause myths you've heard and debunk them with the facts.
- ☐ Research how different cultures view menopause and how it aligns with your experience.
- ☐ Reflect on how the media has portrayed menopause and whether it's accurate or not.
- ☐ Look into the historical views on menopause and how much has changed over the years.
- ☐ Share your new understanding of menopause with others who may hold onto misconceptions.

Action Plan:

1. **Challenge Myths:** Embrace a sense of curiosity and open-mindedness. Write down a few common menopause myths you've encountered and research the facts to debunk them. This process will keep you engaged and interested in the topic.

2. **Cultural Exploration:** Engage in a process of introspection. Learn about how different cultures experience and celebrate menopause and reflect on what you find most interesting. This will make you feel thoughtful and contemplative about the topic.

3. **Media Critique:** Watch or read about how menopause is portrayed in the media and analyze whether it reflects your reality or promotes misconceptions.

4. **Historical Perspective:** Study how views on menopause have evolved over the centuries and note what's changed and what remains the same.

5. **Share Knowledge:** You now have the power of accurate information. Share the facts about menopause with friends, family, or colleagues who might still believe in outdated myths. This will make you feel confident and capable of challenging misconceptions.

18. A New Beginning: Embracing the Next Chapter

"This is the time to redefine what beauty means to you. It's not about how you look, but how you feel and live your life." — Unknown

The menopause is the end of one story and the start of a new one full of chances to grow, learn about yourself and start over. Here's to embracing who you are and living with the confidence and knowledge of getting older. This fresh start isn't just about getting through menopause; it's also about living in the following years.

Rediscovering Yourself.

One of the most liberating aspects of postmenopause is the opportunity to rediscover yourself. After years of being occupied with work, family, and other responsibilities, now is the time to return to the activities that bring you joy. The possibilities are endless; whether you want to explore a new hobby or revive an old one, the choice is entirely yours. This newfound freedom is yours to embrace and enjoy.

Rediscover Your Passion.

Many women think that after menopause is the best time to get interested in old hobbies again. Imagine that you used to love art but haven't picked up a brush in decades. You could also want to start a yard or learn to play the guitar. Now is the time to pursue these interests without anything that might have stopped you in the past. The joy of rediscovering these old passions can bring a sense of nostalgia and excitement.

I felt like making quilts again, so I removed my old sewing machine, which had been stored in the closet for years and dusted it off. The first time I threaded that needle, it felt like seeing an old friend again. The times of day when I sew are some of the calmest and most fun. It is a lesson that the things we love will always be there for us; we must make time for them again.

Try Something New:

At this stage of life, you also have the freedom to explore new experiences. Stepping outside your comfort zone, such as learning a new language, starting yoga, or joining a local theatre group, can be incredibly fulfilling. It keeps your mind and body engaged and can also lead to new friendships and experiences that enrich your life. Embracing these new experiences can make you feel adventurous and open-minded.

A friend of mine started sailing when she was 60 years old. She had never done it before but was always interested in it and now spends her weekends paddling on calm lakes, where she finds peace and connection with nature that she didn't know she needed. It's encouraging to see how trying something new can bring joy in ways you didn't expect.

Old Age And Wisdom: What Menopause Teach Us About Living.

It's not just your body that changes during menopause; your emotions and spirit also change. This stage of life gives you a deep knowledge that you can only get from living. Take some time to think about your past, what you've learned, and how you want to move forward.

Embracing Change:

The most significant lesson that menopause teaches us is how to embrace change. While the physical changes can be daunting, they remind us that life is constantly evolving. Accepting these changes with grace builds resilience that helps us navigate life's unpredictable twists and turns.

At first, I didn't want the changes that came with menopause. Getting older and all the things that came with it made me feel bad. But as time passed, I learned to accept these changes as standard parts of life and not fear them.

This new way of looking at things has also made me more flexible in other areas, like when I must deal with unexpected problems at work or when things change in my personal life.

Appreciating What Matters:

As we age, we often gain clarity about what truly matters. The superficial concerns that once seemed so vital start to fade away, leaving space for what counts: relationships, health, and personal fulfillment. This wisdom allows us to prioritize our time and energy in ways that bring us the most joy and satisfaction.

In retrospect, I used to worry a lot about things that didn't matter, like whether I looked good or was living up to everyone's standards. Now, I pay attention to what makes me healthy and happy. When you let go of old worries, you can focus on what's essential in life.

How To Have The Best Life Postmenopause.

To live your best life postmenopause, you need to do more than deal with your symptoms. It would help if you excelled in all areas of your life. Take advantage of this time by following these suggestions.

Make Your Health A Priority.

As you age, taking charge of your health becomes increasingly important. A balanced diet, regular exercise, and medical check-ups are vital to maintaining vitality. Equally significant is nurturing your mental well-being. Engaging in activities that bring you joy, practicing mindfulness, and spending time with loved ones can all contribute to your mental sharpness and overall happiness. This empowerment allows you to lead a fulfilling life postmenopause with confidence and control, knowing that you are actively shaping your well-being.

Embrace the Joy of Daily Activities.

Make a conscious effort to incorporate activities that bring joy into your daily routine. Whether spending time with your grandkids, engaging in a hobby or reading a good book, these moments of happiness make life truly fulfilling. Remember, life is too short not to include joy in your daily activities.

Stay Connected: The Power of Community.

Building and maintaining friendships is a key component of a happy life, especially as we age. Don't hesitate to meet new people, stay in touch with family and friends, and join clubs or groups that interest you. The community can provide you with the support, friendship, and sense of belonging essential for a fulfilling life postmenopause.

Joining a book club was one of the best things I did after menopause. Along with talking about great books, it put me in touch with a great group of women who have become close friends. These individuals play a significant role in my life now. I can't picture it without them.

Travel And Adventure: Exploring the World with New Eyes.

Traveling is another great thing about life; postmenopause is the best time to see the world through fresh eyes. Travel can be a source of inspiration and renewal, whether to go to a dream place, take a spontaneous road trip, or explore your neighborhood.

Seeing The World In Another Way.

Now that you're getting older, traveling can be very different from when you were younger. You may become more aware of the world's beauty and variety and more interested in the histories and cultures of the places you visit. Traveling isn't just about checking places off a list; it's about living each moment to the fullest.

Solo Traveling.

Some people look forward to traveling alone postmenopause. Going to new places by yourself, at your own pace, and based on what interests you can be very powerful. Traveling by yourself can also help you think about yourself and grow as a person. It's a chance to be adventurous and daring, to explore the world on your terms, and to feel the liberating sense of freedom that comes with solo travel.

I went on my first trip by myself, postmenopause, and it was one of the best times of my life. I went to Italy, a place I had always wanted to see. I spent my days exploring art museums, drinking espresso in bars, and enjoying the beautiful scenery. When I traveled alone, I felt free to do whatever I wanted, whenever I wanted. When I returned home, I felt more independent and surer of myself.

Going On Adventures with family or friends.

Going on trips can also be a great way to get closer to family and friends. Shared new experiences can make memories that last a lifetime, whether a family holiday with people of all ages or a trip with a group of friends.

Legacy And Reflection: Leaving Your Mark.

Thinking about what you want to leave behind as you start this new stage is normal. Legacy and reflection are about considering the impact you want to have on the world and the people around you. It isn't always about significant actions or accomplishments; it's about how you affect the people around you and the world.

Reflecting On Your Life.

Take some time to reflect on your life's journey and the lessons you've learned. Which experiences bring you the greatest happiness? What insights have you gained about yourself and your environment? Reflecting on your experiences can provide a sense of calm and satisfaction, helping you appreciate how far you've come and the person you've become postmenopause. This journey of self-discovery is an integral part of living a fulfilling life postmenopause.

Giving Back.

A lot of women think that postmenopause is the best time to help others. It can be very satisfying to give back, whether it's through teaching, volunteering, or supporting causes that are important to you. You can use your knowledge and experience to improve the world and, in doing so, feel a deep sense of purpose and satisfaction.

Since retiring, helping at a neighborhood food bank has been one of the best things I've ever done. I feel connected and like I'm making a change in my neighborhood, which gives me a sense of purpose.

Making A Difference.

It's not just the things you leave behind but how you live your life daily. Your love and kindness, the knowledge you share, and the memories you have make life worth living. If you live with meaning and purpose, you can leave a memory that shows the best of who you are.

Thinking about my heritage, I understand it's not about the things I've done or the things I'll leave behind. It's about building connections, sharing love, and affecting the people in my life. That is what matters most.

Accepting the next part of your life after menopause means getting to know yourself again, living wisely, and finding joy in new things. You should think about your journey, give back, and leave a memory that shows who you are. Now is the time to grow, discover, and live a life full of love and meaning.

Focus on Your Legacy.

Reflect on what legacy you want to leave behind. This could involve family, community, or creative pursuits. Ask yourself how you want to be remembered and what impact you wish to make moving forward.

Practice Self-Compassion: Be kind to yourself as you enter this new phase. Aging can bring challenges, but it also offers unique rewards. Celebrate your accomplishments, embrace your wisdom, and take pride in all you've become.

Checklist:

- ☐ Acknowledge the end of menopause and the start of a new phase in your life.
- ☐ Reflect on how menopause has changed you emotionally, mentally, and physically.
- ☐ Explore new passions, hobbies, or personal goals post-menopause.
- ☐ Embrace the wisdom and life experience gained through this transition.
- ☐ Recognize that post-menopause offers opportunities for growth, self-discovery, and reinvention.
- ☐ Prioritize long-term health goals, including physical, emotional, and mental well-being.

Action Plan:

1. **Reflect on Your Menopause Journey:** Take time to journal your experiences during menopause. What have you learned about yourself? How have you grown? Acknowledge the challenges you've faced and the resilience you've shown. Don't hesitate to seek professional help if you find it particularly challenging. You've come a long way; your journey is a testament to your strength and resilience.

2. **Set New Personal Goals:** With menopause behind you, excitedly, look forward to this next chapter. Whether learning a new skill, traveling, or engaging in a new hobby, list specific goals that excite you and bring purpose to your life. These goals will give you a sense of direction and purpose as you embark on this new phase of your life.

3. **Nurture Your Health:** Commit to long-term self-care. This could include scheduling regular check-ups, starting or maintaining an exercise routine, and staying mindful of your diet to support bone and heart health in post-menopause. Your well-being is your most fantastic resource. Taking care of your health is a way of showing love and respect for yourself.

4. **Rediscover Old Passions:** Think about activities or hobbies you may have put on the back burner during your busy years of work and family life. Now is the time to revisit those passions and explore new ones.

5. **Stay Socially Connected:** Build or maintain a support system of friends, family, or groups that uplift you. Consider joining a book club, volunteering at a local charity, or participating in a hobby group. If your loved ones are far away, you can stay connected through regular phone calls, video chats, or even by writing letters. These days, technology makes it easier than ever to keep in touch. Being socially active and connecting with like-minded individuals can help you feel fulfilled and supported.

6. **Explore New Adventures:** Whether it's travel or new experiences close to home, consider how you can embrace a spirit of adventure. Make a list of places you've always wanted to visit or experiences you've dreamed of trying—then start planning!

7. **Focus on Your Legacy:** Reflect on what legacy you want to leave behind. This could involve family, community, or creative pursuits. Ask yourself how you want to be remembered and what impact you wish to make moving forward.

8. **Practice Self-Compassion:** Be kind to yourself as you enter this new phase. Aging can bring challenges, but it also offers unique rewards. Celebrate your accomplishments, embrace your wisdom, and take pride in all you've become.

Conclusion: You've Got This!

ow that you've successfully navigated menopause and beyond, it's a moment to pause and reflect on the incredible strength of our collective journey. Menopause is often perceived as a challenging phase, marked by hot flashes, mood swings, and changes in body shape, but it's also a time of significant personal growth and transformation.

We've weathered these physical and emotional changes together, emerging stronger, wiser, and more resilient. Whether it's the newfound confidence to speak up for your needs or the resilience to adapt to physical changes, take pride in our shared journey and the women we've become.

Reflecting On Your Menopausal Journey: The Woman You've Become.

As you reflect on your menopausal journey, it's important to thank the woman you've become for the strength, resilience, and knowledge she has obtained. Take a moment to journal about your experiences, the challenges you've overcome, and the lessons you've learned. Consider writing about a particularly challenging moment and how you overcame it or a lesson you learned about self-care during this time. This will help you appreciate the growth and transformation that has taken place.

More In-Depth Knowledge Of Yourself.

Learning so much about yourself on this trip is one of the most essential things it's taught you. You've had to deal with changes that may have seemed too much at times, but they've helped you learn more about who you are. While going through menopause, you may face hurdles that help you see your authentic self more clearly. You probably know your needs, wants and limits better now. Being more self-aware is helpful as you move forward.

Slowing down and paying attention to my body and mind became crucial during menopause. I had to abandon some old habits and standards, which wasn't always easy, but it's helped me become much more aware of what I need to be healthy and happy. It's like meeting an old friend again but with more kindness and understanding this time.

Appreciating The Change.

In ways you might not have thought possible, menopause teaches you how to accept change. Sometimes, the changes in your body, like hot flashes or weight gain or loss, can be annoying, but they also force you to adapt and find new ways to live that work for you.

For instance, you might have had to change your diet or exercise routine to manage weight changes or find new ways to manage stress to reduce the frequency of hot flashes. This skill of being able to change helps you in all parts of your life by making you more open to new things.

I remember having a hard time with my body's sudden changes — nothing worked as it used to! But I saw that fighting these changes wasn't working overtime. Instead, I learned to change and find better ways to eat, work out, and dress. You'll find so much peace when you stop fighting the new you and start accepting it.

Celebrate Your Incredible Strength.

Take a moment to think about how strong you are to get through menopause. Not only do you have to deal with the symptoms, but you also must keep living your life, working, caring for others, and doing the things you love. You should be proud of how strong you are like that.

A Final Note: Celebrating Your Strength and Resilience.

Remember to honor the strength and toughness that got you to this point as you move on to the next part of your life. At menopause, women often feel like they've lost something—their youth, their fertility, or their energy. But at the same time, they gain a lot. You're more intelligent, more confident, and better understand who you are now. You now know how to put your health first, speak up for what you need, and enjoy the changes in this stage of life.

How To Find Joy In The New You.

Embrace the new you with joy and peace. You've earned the right to live on your terms, doing what brings you happiness and letting go of what no longer serves you. Find joy in this new phase by exploring new experiences, spending quality time with loved ones, or simply relishing the tranquility of self-acceptance. Consider treating yourself to a spa day, planning a trip to a place you've always wanted to visit, or starting a new hobby to celebrate the new you. This is a time for joy and new beginnings.

Since I went through menopause, the little things that used to make me sad now bring me a lot of joy. I value these times more now, whether it's a quiet morning with a cup of tea, a long walk in the park, or a weekend with my family. Some people are happy knowing who they are and what's important to them. I remember feeling lost and confused during menopause, but I also remember the joy and peace that came with accepting the changes and embracing the new me.

Resilience As Your Superpower.

Your resilience is not just a quality; it's your superpower. You've conquered the challenges of menopause, and that same strength will guide you through any future obstacles. It's about bouncing back after a setback; each experience makes you more resilient and capable. You've proven to yourself that you can handle whatever life throws your way, and that's something to be genuinely proud of. You are strong, capable, and ready for whatever comes next.

Sometimes, I thought I couldn't handle another hot flash, another night of being unable to sleep, or another angry outburst. Despite that, I always got through it. Each time, I felt stronger and better able to handle things. I am prepared to confront whatever challenges arise next.

Living With Purpose.

Stay focused on living a meaningful life as you go. Now that you know more, make decisions that align with your morals and goals. Let the strong, tough woman you've become show through in your relationships, work, and personal   life.

Finally, You Can Do This!

It may have been a wild ride through menopause, but you got through it with style, fun, and strength. Accept that you can do anything as you move on to the next part of your life. It was one of the most complicated changes a woman can go through, but you made it through it more vital than ever.

Cheers to the amazing woman you've become, your trip, and your fantastic future. You can do it!

Helpful Links And More Reading.

This chapter equips you with the tools and information to take charge of your menopause journey. It instills in you the confidence to navigate this phase with grace, fun, and strength. Remember, now is the time to prioritize your health and well-being. You are capable of this!

Where to Find Out More:

Menopause can feel like wandering in a dense forest without a plan. But fear not; there are numerous supportive tools out there to guide you through this process.

Books:

- **"The Wisdom of Menopause" book by Dr. Christiane Northrup.** It's like having a wise friend who has been through everything. Dr. Northrup looks at menopause from various angles, combining medical knowledge with mental and emotional health.

- **The book "Menopause Confidential" by Dr. Tara Allmen.** This book tells you about the science behind menopause and is easy to understand. It also has some fun parts to keep things light.

- **Hillary Wright and Elizabeth Ward's "The Menopause Diet Plan".**

  If you're looking to control your symptoms through food, this book is full of valuable tips, meal plans, and tasty recipes that are perfect for women going through menopause.

Websites:

- The Menopause Society **– Formerly Called North American Menopause Society (NAMS).**

  This site is a treasure trove of information. It has the latest study, expert tips, and a valuable tool for tracking menopause symptoms.

- Menopause Matters:

  This site is based in the UK and has information on everything from signs to treatments. It also has a forum where women going through the same things can meet with each other.

- My Menopause Doctor:

  This site, run by Dr. Louise Newson, provides easy-to-read information based on evidence about hormone replacement therapy, lifestyle changes, and other menopause-related topics.

Helpful Groups:

- <u>Red Hot Mamas</u>: It is one of the country's most extensive teaching programs about menopause. It offers many tools and support groups, both online and in person.

- <u>Menopause Support Group On Facebook</u>: This is an active, private Facebook group for menopausal women. It's a place where they can share their stories, ask questions, and get help — like having a group of women going through menopause right at their fingertips.

Recommended Health And Wellness Practitioners: Finding The Right Help.

It's like assembling a dream team of health and fitness professionals to guide you through menopause. Whether you need a doctor who understands it, a nutritionist who can navigate the hormonal ups and downs, or a therapist who can help you manage the mental ups and downs, knowing where to start is crucial.

- **<u>Gynecologists:</u>** Choose a gynecologist who specializes in menopause or is qualified by The Menopause Society, formerly North American Menopause Society (NAMS). They will empower you with the most up-to-date treatments and can help you weigh the pros and cons of choices like HRT.

- **<u>Endocrinologists:</u>** If your symptoms are linked to hormones, an endocrinologist can help you understand what's happening in your body and manage your treatments, relieving you.

- **<u>Therapists And Counselors:</u>** A therapist who focuses on women's health or changes in midlife can be beneficial. Cognitive behavioral therapy (CBT) has been shown to help with mood changes, anxiety, and sadness that come with menopause.

- **<u>Nutritionists And Dietitians:</u>** Look for a nutritionist who knows how to help women going through menopause. They can help you develop a diet that supports your changing your body, protects your bones and heart, and stops those hot flashes.

- **<u>Physical Therapists:</u>** They specialize in women's health, especially those who offer pelvic floor treatment, can make a big difference in your sexual health and happiness.

Documenting Your Menopause Journey.

Making a record of your menopause journey, such as writing in a journal, can be a powerful tool to help you deal with the changes that come with menopause.

It provides a safe space to vent, reflect, and keep track of your progress. It's not just about documenting your journey but also about understanding and managing it. You might also find it interesting to see how far you've come.

Consequently, it would help if you tried out the following:

- **Symptom Tracker:** You can better understand your body's changes by diligently noting your concerns daily or weekly. This knowledge can empower you, instilling a strong sense of control and confidence in managing your menopausal journey.

- **Mood Journal:** Simultaneously noting your symptoms and emotions can help you see the link between physical symptoms like hot flashes and emotional changes like mood swings. This practice can foster a deeper awareness and understanding of your body's responses.

- **Gratitude List:** Each day, list three things that you appreciate. These could be simple things like a good night's sleep, a delicious meal, or a supportive friend. For instance, you could enjoy the comfort of your bed, the taste of your favorite meal, or the understanding of a friend.

Focusing on the good things in your life can help you maintain a positive outlook and deal with the problems that come with menopause. This practice of gratitude can boost your mental well-being by shifting your focus from the challenges of menopause to the positive aspects of your life.

Menopausal Journaling Prompts.

The following prompts guide your reflection, foster self-awareness, and provide a space for both the challenges and the positive transformations that menopause can bring. They are self-discovery tools, helping you delve deeper into your thoughts and feelings during this significant life transition. Using these prompts, you can better understand your menopause journey and learn to manage it more effectively.

- **"Which was the most significant symptom of menopause for me, and how did I react towards it?"** - *You might understand your menopause journey better if you think back to how you felt at the start.*

....

....

....

....

....

....

- **"What symptoms affect me the most, and what strategies do I use to manage them?"** - *Understanding your problems is the first thing you need to do to find solutions.*

....

....

....

....

....

....

- **"How has menopause changed the way I think about getting older and being a woman?"** - *After reading this question, Consider how you see yourself and your life.*

....

....

....

....

....

....

- **"What types of self-care have been the most helpful for me during this time?"** - *This question makes you feel valuable and important by highlighting how important it is to take care of yourself. Enjoying your wins, even if they are small, can be beneficial.*

....
....
....
....
....
....

- **"How has my relationship with my body changed during menopause?"** - *Reflect on the physical changes you're experiencing. How do you feel about them, and how can you nurture a more positive relationship with your body?*

....
....
....
....
....
....

- **"What menopausal experiences most often affect me, and what messages might they be conveying to me?"** - *Uncover the feelings you go through throughout menopause — be it frustration, depression, or happiness? What patterns do you notice, and how can you healthily process them?*

....

....

....

....

....

....

- **"What are three things I've learned about myself through this menopause journey?"** - *Write about the personal insights menopause has given you. What strengths or characteristics have come to light during this transition?*

....

....

....

....

....

....

- **"What everyday activities or self-care practices enable me to feel my most radiant throughout menopause?"** - *This question underscores the importance of self-care. It's a reminder that caring for yourself is not a luxury but a necessity. You can feel valued and important by prioritizing these practices, boosting your self-esteem and well-being.*

....
....
....
....
....
....

- **"How has menopause influenced my close relationships and social events?"** - *Think back on how your social life could have changed and examine what you need from your support system. Have certain friendships strengthened, or have others faded?*

....
....
....
....
....
....

- **"What activities allow me to connect with myself and bring joy?"** - *Take note of the things or tasks you enjoy. How can you prioritize these to maintain a sense of fulfillment and pleasure?*

....

....

....

....

....

....

- **"What's one fear or concern I have about menopause, and how can I address it?"** - *Examine any specific fears about menopause (e.g., aging, health, relationships) and brainstorm steps to tackle them head-on.*

....

....

....

....

....

....

- **"How do I define beauty for myself at this stage in life?"** - *Thinking about how your sense of beauty has changed. How has going through menopause altered the way you feel about your looks, and how can you accept new ideas of what is beautiful?*

....

....

....

....

....

....

- **"How has menopause influenced my spiritual or personal growth?"**- *Consider how this transition might have opened new paths for inner growth. What practices, beliefs, or shifts have you noticed in your spiritual or personal development?*

....

....

....

....

....

....

- **"What good qualities or characteristics become obvious during my menopausal journey?"** - *Pay attention to the advantages of menopause and aging. What wisdom, patience, or resilience have you gained, and how can you continue to nurture those traits?*

....

....

....

....

....

....

A Guide to Some Of the Good Products for Menopausal Women.

Rest assured, there are numerous effective products on the market designed to alleviate the symptoms of menopause. With their proven track record of efficacy, these options can bring a sense of relief and significantly improve your quality of life, giving you the confidence to manage your symptoms effectively.

- <u>**Cooling Products:**</u> If you have hot flashes or night sweats, you might want to buy cooling pillows, bed sheets, and fans. Products from brands like *Chillow* and *BedJet* are made to keep you cool and comfy.

These products range in price, so it's important to consider your budget when purchasing. However, it's important to note that excessive use of cooling products can lead to health issues, so it's best to use them in moderation.

- **<u>Vaginal Moisturizers And Lubricants:</u>** Not many people like to talk about vaginal dryness, but it happens to a lot of people. Hormone-free choices that keep your skin moist for a long time include **Replens** and **Yes**.

  However, it's important to consult your doctor before using these products, as they may not be suitable for everyone and could cause allergic reactions or other health issues.

- **<u>Menopause Supplements:</u>** Supplements like **Evening Primrose Oil, Black Cohosh**, and **Red Clover** are commonly used to manage menopausal symptoms.

  However, it's crucial to consult your doctor before introducing any new substance to your regimen. This responsible approach ensures its safety and suitability for your unique health needs, providing you with a sense of security and confidence in your choices.

- **<u>Tools For Mind And Body:</u>** Check out apps like **Headspace** or **Calm** for guided meditation and calm routines. Yoga mats and bolsters are other tools that can help you incorporate mind-body routines into your daily life.

- **<u>Exercise Equipment:</u>** Strength training is vital in maintaining bone health during menopause. By investing in tools such as ***dumbbells***, ***exercise bands***, and a ***yoga mat***, you can empower yourself to take control of your health and well-being. Regular exercise is not just vital, it's empowering, helping you manage menopausal symptoms and maintain overall health.

About the Author.

Hey there! I'm Avery Rodriguez. Just like many of you, I'm on this journey through menopause. I'm not a doctor, a scientist, or a famous health expert. I'm just a regular woman who's had her fair share of hot flashes, mood swings, and late-night Google searches. I wrote this book because I know how it feels to be in your shoes, and I want you to know that you're not alone.

When I first started this journey, I was overwhelmed by medical terms, conflicting advice, and the dismissive *just deal with it* attitude. I wanted to learn more and share what I had found in a way that felt like talking with a friend over coffee (or wine because, let's be honest, some days call for it). My goal was to provide information and offer valuable insights that help you feel informed, empowered, and confident in navigating this journey. Rest assured, the content in this book is backed by reliable sources, thorough research and personal experiences.

Sharing My Story: My Journey Through Menopause.

My journey through menopause didn't start with a bang. It was more of a whisper that became a shout overtime. I remember being soaked in sweat when I woke up in the middle of the night for the first time. *"Did I leave the heat on?"* was the initial thought that entered my mind. When these sweating fits at night started happening all the time, I knew something bigger was happening.

Early menopause hit me when I was in my late 40s, and it was a wild ride. In one moment, I was crying over an ad for dog food, and in the next, I was yelling at my husband for breathing too loudly. Not only did the mental ups and downs throw me off, but so did the changes in my body. For some reason, my pants wouldn't zip up, and I felt like I was living in a world where everything was moving at lightning speed.

But I discovered something unique through it all. Menopause, in a way, is both an end and a beginning. It's a time to pause, reflect, and redefine what's important. It's messy, hard to understand, and sometimes downright annoying, but it's also a chance to start anew, learn from our past, and live our lives on our terms. It's a transformative journey that offers hope and a fresh perspective. I want to share with you that it's possible to come out of this experience stronger, wiser, and more in tune with yourself.

That's why I'm here telling you, my story. I understand your situation because I have experienced it as well. I found it helpful to write this book, and I hope you find it useful to read it. Let's get through this maze with a bit of fun, a lot of kindness, and the knowledge that we're not going through this alone. I also encourage you to share your own experiences and insights, as this book is not just about my journey, but about our collective journey through menopause.